Joggin' Your Noggin

Challenging Word Activities for Seniors

Volume Three

Mary Randolph, MS, CCC

Speech-Language Pathologist

Published by
Noggin Joggin' Books
Easton, CT 06612

ISBN:1480023760
ISBN-13:978-1480023765

ACKNOWLEDGEMENTS

With appreciation to family and friends, and especially to my husband, Paul, for his support and encouragement in publishing Volume Three.

Likewise, with continued gratitude to my brother, Joe, for his assistance in preparing this third book in the series.

And to Microsoft Office Online for use of clip art that adds so much to the cover and interior of the books.

INTRODUCTION

This third book in the series introduces several new word games, while retaining much of the popular format presented in prior issues. Samples of the latest challenges include:

- Name the Activity
- Name the Synonym
- Identify the Action or Use of an Object
- Name the Occupation, Given "Tools of the Trade"
- Name the Food or Drink, Given its Ingredients
- Identify the Famous Location

All tasks are carefully designed to challenge the minds of seniors, particularly those in mild to moderate stages of Alzheimer's disease. Answers are provided on the page following each game for easy accessibility. Readers may complete the activity books independently, or along with a family member, friend or caregiver. Activity directors may engage a group of participants in nursing homes or assisted living facilities. Regardless of the setting, all will enjoy reminiscing, laughing, sensing the pride of success or simply appreciating the moment.

A retired speech-language pathologist, the author has over twenty years of experience in helping adults and children faced with memory, thinking and word-finding deficits. Many approaches used in speech therapy are incorporated in the word games found in the series. These include the use of sound and context cues, visualization, fill-in's, and opposites. For example, when a word slips our mind, we can often recall it by thinking of its initial sound or letter. Similarly, our memory is sometimes jogged by picturing what a person or place looks like or what we do with a particular object. Or we might use the "fill-in-the-blank" technique. For example, I might not remember the name of my cousin in California. But if I say, "I went to California to visit _____," the person's name may pop up! Another technique is the use of an opposite; for example, "It's not morning; it's _____."

Many language drills, such as rapid naming and categorization, also improve retrieval ability. Some of the games may seem easy to complete; others may present considerable challenge. Regardless of the level of difficulty, the activities provide essential calisthenics for the brain to help maintain and improve memory and word-finding skills.

TABLE OF CONTENTS

This book is comprised of four chapters, each with the same 20 games. Answers are provided on the page directly following each game.

Game	Game Title	Page #
1	Circle Items in a Category	1/2, 41/42, 81/82, 121/122
2	Name Items in a Category	3/4, 43/44, 83/84, 123/124
3	Name a Category	5/6, 45/46, 85/86, 125/126
4	Focus on One Topic and Fill in the Blank, Given the first Letter	7/8, 47/48, 87/88, 127/128
5	Identify the Word that Doesn't Belong	9/10, 49/50, 89/90, 129/130
6	Fill in the Blank, Given a Clue and the First Letter	11/12, 51/52, 91/92, 131/132

TABLE OF CONTENTS (CONT'D)

Game	Game Title	Page #
7	Unscramble a Word, Given the Category	13/14, 53/54, 93/94, 133/134
8	Picture a Description and Name the Word	15/16, 55/56, 95/96, 135/136
9	Complete the Common Saying	17/18, 57/58, 97/98, 137/138
10	Name the Synonym	19/20, 59/60 99/100, 139/140
11	Identify the Action or Use of the Object	21/22 61/62, 101/102, 141/142
12	Name the Activity	23/24, 63/64 103/104, 143/144
13	Name the Occupation, Given "Tools of the Trade"	25/26, 65/66, 105/106, 145/146

TABLE OF CONTENTS (CONT'D)

Game	Game Title	Page #
14	Name the Food or Drink, Given its Ingredients	27/28, 67/68, 107/108, 147/148
15	Identify the Famous Location	29/30, 69/70, 109/110, 149/150
16	Fill In the Person	31/32, 71/72, 111/112, 151/152
17	Fill In the Object	33/34, 73/74, 113/114, 153/154
18	Fill In the Place	35/36, 75/76, 115/116, 155/156
19	Fill In the Blank - Time or Event	37/38, 77/78, 117/118, 157/158
20	Fill In the Blank - Reason	39/40, 79/80, 119/120, 159/160

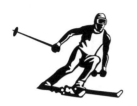

> **CIRCLE** the **WINTER OLYMPIC SPORTS** that appear on the 3 lists below. You should find 12 sports all together. Good luck!

List 1	List 2	List 3
swimming	diving	sailing
luge	equestrian	Alpine skiing
archery	snowboarding	rowing
diving	field hockey	volleyball
badminton	fencing	speed skating
figure skating	freestyle skiing	cross country skiing
boxing	gymnastics	ice hockey
bowling	Nordic combined	croquet
canoeing	water polo	tennis
cycling	bobsleigh	shooting
curling	wrestling	ski jumping

ANSWERS TO:
CIRCLE 12 WINTER
OLYMPIC SPORTS

List 1	List 2	List 3
luge		Alpine skiing /
	snowboarding /	
		speed skating
figure skating /	freestyle skiing /	cross country skiing
		ice hockey
	Nordic combined	
	bobsleigh /	
curling		ski jumping /

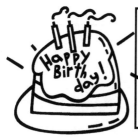

NAME 10 THINGS
you might see at a
CHILD'S BIRTHDAY PARTY.
HINT: Think of decorations, food
and games.

1. _____

2. _____

3. _____

4. _____

5. _____

6. _____

7. _____

8. _____

9. _____

10. _____

ANSWERS TO:
10 THINGS
you might see at a
CHILD'S BIRTHDAY PARTY.

---

1.   cake

2.   candles

3.   cupcakes

4.   balloons

5.   streamers

6.   hats

7.   horns

8.   gifts

9.   games

10.   goody bags

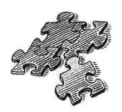

> **READ** the **ITEMS**; then **NAME** the **CATEGORY**. For example, "dog, cat, bird, goldfish and hamster" go together because they belong to the category of "pets."

ITEMS	CATEGORY
dog, cat, bird, goldfish, hamster	pets
respiratory, digestive, circulatory, endocrine, reproductive	BREATHING
hot, cold, tepid, warm, freezing	WEATHER
hat, helmet, cap, bonnet, sombrero	HEAD WEAR
Yosemite, Acadia, Yellowstone, Glacier, Grand Canyon	NATIONAL PARKS
jacks, blocks, marbles, pick-up-sticks	GAMES
measuring cups and spoons, bowls, mixer, spatula, pan	COOKING
rain, snow, hail, drizzle, sleet	WEATHER
biceps, triceps, flexors, trapezius, quadriceps	BODY PARTS

ANSWERS TO: NAME the CATEGORY.

ITEMS	CATEGORY
dog, cat, bird, goldfish, hamster	pets
respiratory, digestive, circulatory, endocrine, reproductive	body systems
hot, cold, tepid, warm, freezing	water temperatures
hat, helmet, cap, bonnet, sombrero	headwear
Yosemite, Acadia, Yellowstone, Glacier, Grand Canyon	national parks
jacks, blocks, marbles, pick-up-sticks	old-time toys
measuring cups and spoons, bowls, mixer, spatula, pan	baking implements
rain, snow, hail, drizzle, sleet	precipitation
biceps, triceps, flexors, trapezius, quadriceps	muscles

$$$ | **FOCUS** on **MONEY** and **FILL IN** the **BLANK.**

1. If you need help filing tax returns, hire an _a_____

2. The US coin valued at 25 cents is a _q_____

3. One of the safest investments, because of backing by the US government, is a savings _b_____

4. When people purchase stocks or bonds, expecting to make a profit, they make a financial _i_____

5. Lottery winnings, or an unexpected inheritance, are types of _w_____

6. When you put the blame on someone else, you are said to "Pass the _b_____ "

7. The legal document used to pass property upon death is called a _w_____

8. Employers pay their employees a wage or _s_____

9. When you pay a very high price for something, you "Pay through the _n_____ "

10. Unscramble these words (related to money):

   N A C F I N E S   _____

   E T W H A L   _____

   S N T E C   _____

   V R P E Y T O   _____

   C O N C A U T   _____

ANSWERS TO:
FOCUS on MONEY

1. If you need help filing tax returns, hire an _accountant_

2. The US coin valued at 25 cents is a _quarter_

3. One of the safest investments, because of backing by the US government, is a savings _bond_

4. When people purchase stocks or bonds, expecting to make a profit, they make a financial _investment_

5. Lottery winnings, or an unexpected inheritance, are types of _windfalls_

6. When you put the blame on someone else, you are said to "Pass the _buck_ "

7. The legal document used to pass property upon death is called a _will_

8. Employers pay their employees a wage or _salary_

9. When you pay a very high price for something, you "Pay through the _nose_ "

10. Unscramble these words (related to money):

N A C F I N E S	_finances_
E T W H A L	_wealth_
S N T E C	_cents_
V R P E Y T O	_poverty_
C O N C A U T	_account_

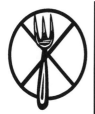

> **FILL IN** the **BOX** with the **WORD THAT DOESN'T BELONG.** For example, "dog, cat, goldfish and hamster" are all pets; "fork" is NOT a pet—it doesn't belong in the group.

ITEMS	DOESN'T BELONG
dog, cat, fork, goldfish, hamster	fork
sister, mother, aunt, uncle, grandmother	UNCLE
red, yellow, blue, purple	PURPLE
ugly, lovely, gorgeous, beautiful, pretty	UGLY
fast, quick, lethargic, speedy, swift	LETHARGIC
pauper, beggar, hobo, heiress, vagabond	HEIRESS
car, helicopter, truck, van, motorcycle	HELICOPTOR
radio, magazine, book, newspaper, journal	RADIO
chicken, turkey, quail, duck, robin	ROBIN
drum, cymbals, tambourine, bells, clarinet	BELLS

ANSWERS TO: THE WORD THAT <u>DOESN'T</u> <u>BELONG</u>.

<u>ITEMS</u>	<u>DOESN'T BELONG</u>
dog, cat, fork, goldfish, hamster	fork
sister, mother, aunt, uncle, grandmother	uncle
red, yellow, blue, purple	purple
ugly, lovely, gorgeous, beautiful, pretty	ugly
fast, quick, lethargic, speedy, swift	lethargic
pauper, beggar, hobo, heiress, vagabond	heiress
car, helicopter, truck, van, motorcycle	helicopter
radio, magazine, book, newspaper, journal	radio
chicken, turkey, quail, duck, robin	robin
drum, cymbals, tambourine, bells, clarinet	clarinet

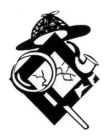

Use the clues to help you
NAME the **WORD**.

1. A dish made with noodles, meatballs and tomato sauce	S _ _ _ _ _ _ _ _
2. A green vegetable associated with strong muscles	S _ _ _ _ _ _
3. A three-dimensional model of the earth	G _ _ _ _
4. A type of heavy equipment used to move the earth	B _ _ _ _ _ _ _
5. A wild cat with black stripes	T _ _ _ _
6. The material of elephant tusks used for art and manufacturing	I _ _ _ _
7. A type of nut eaten by squirrels	A _ _ _ _
8. The forest animal with a reputation for being very sly	F _ _
9. The tool used to hang laundry on a line to dry	C _ _ _ _ _ _ _ _
10. A clothing fastener that fits through a hole	B _ _ _ _ _

> **ANSWERS TO:**
> Use the clues to help you
> **NAME** the **WORD**.

1. A dish made with noodles, meatballs and tomato sauce	**spaghetti**
2. A green vegetable associated with strong muscles	**spinach**
3. A three-dimensional model of the earth	**globe**
4. A type of heavy equipment used to move the earth	**bulldozer**
5. A wild cat with black stripes	**tiger**
6. The material of elephant tusks used for art and manufacturing	**ivory**
7. A type of nut eaten by squirrels	**acorn**
8. The forest animal with a reputation for being very sly	**fox**
9. The tool used to hang laundry on a line to dry	**clothespin**
10. A clothing fastener that fits through a hole	**button**

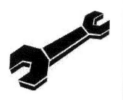

UNSCRAMBLE the
LETTERS to make a word.
HINT: All of the words are
TOOLS. The first one is done
for you.

ENWCRH   W R E N C H

MAMHRE   H _ _ _ _ _

CKHWASA   H _ _ _ _ _ _

LLIRD   D _ _ _ _

LIESPR   P _ _ _ _ _

VELEL   L _ _ _ _

NRSADE   S _ _ _ _ _

REUOTR   R _ _ _ _ _

RIDGNER   G _ _ _ _ _ _

SCHLEI   C _ _ _ _ _

ANSWERS TO:
UNSCRAMBLE the
LETTERS to make a word.

E N W C R H   WRENCH

M A M H R E   HAMMER

C K H W A S A   HACKSAW

L L I R D   DRILL

L I E S P R   PLIERS

V E L E L   LEVEL

N R S A D E   SANDER

R E U O T R   ROUTER

R I D G N E R   GRINDER

S C H L E I   CHISEL

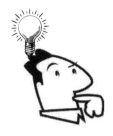

PICTURE the DESCRIPTION; then FILL IN the BLANK.

1. I am a long legged, pink bird that often stands on one leg. I am a _____

2. I am a beautiful fragrant flower, the symbol of love. I am a _____

3. I am a glittering expensive gemstone often seen in engagement rings. I am a _____

4. I am a special type of protective eye covering worn by scuba divers. I am a _____

5. I am a large, mostly white bird, with a long beak and throat pouch to catch fish. I am a _____

6. I am a protective metal suit worn by knights in days of old. I am _____

7. I am a fierce swordsman who fought lions and entertained audiences during the Roman Empire. I am a

_____

8. I am a sport played on ice in which a puck is hit with a stick into a goal. I am _____

9. I am a large board used to ride the waves. I am a

_____

10. I am strips of potatoes, deep fried in oil and often served with ketchup. I am _____

ANSWERS TO:
PICTURE the DESCRIPTION

1. I am a long legged, pink bird that often stands on one leg. I am a _____flamingo_____

2. I am a beautiful fragrant flower, the symbol of love. I am a ___rose___

3. I am a glittering expensive gemstone often seen in engagement rings. I am a __diamond__

4. I am a special type of protective eye covering worn by scuba divers. I am a ___mask___

5. I am a large, mostly white bird, with a long beak and throat pouch to catch fish. I am a _pelican_

6. I am a protective metal suit worn by knights in days of old. I am _armor_

7. I am a fierce swordsman who fought lions and entertained audiences during the Roman Empire. I am a ___gladiator___

8. I am a sport played on ice in which a puck is hit with a stick into a goal. I am ___ice hockey___

9. I am a large board used to ride the waves. I am a ___surfboard___

10. I am strips of potatoes, deep fried in oil and often served with ketchup. I am _French fries_

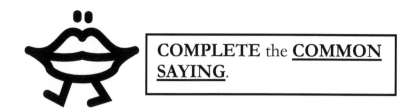

COMPLETE the **COMMON SAYING**.

1. After a draught, rivers might be described as being "as dry as a _____"

2. If you find someone or something difficult to accept, you might say "they're hard to _____"

3. A person who is a disgrace to his family might be described as "a black_____"

4. A person who is very attentive and eager to hear something "is all _____"

5. Someone's favorite (sweetheart) is the "apple of their _____"

6. People who stay up late are called "night _____"

7. A ballet dancer may be described as being "as graceful as a _____"

8. When you recover from sickness or trouble, you are "back on your _____"

9. When a car is almost worn out, it is said to be "on its last _____"

10. If you really irritate or bother someone, they may tell you to "get out of my _____"

ANSWERS TO: COMPLETE the COMMON SAYING.

1. After a draught, rivers might be described as being "as dry as a ___bone___ "
2. If you find someone or something difficult to accept, you might say "they're hard to _stomach_ "
3. A person who is a disgrace to his family might be described as "a black___sheep___ "
4. A person who is very attentive and eager to hear something "is all ___ears___ "
5. Someone's favorite (sweetheart) is the "apple of their ___eye___ "
6. People who stay up late are called "night ___owls___ "
7. A ballet dancer may be described as being "as graceful as a ___swan___ "
8. When you recover from sickness or trouble, you are "back on your ___feet___ "
9. When a car is almost worn out, it is said to be "on its last ___legs___ "
10. If you really irritate or bother someone, they may tell you to "get out of my ___face___ "

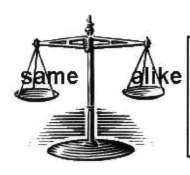

FILL IN the box with a **SYNONYM,** a word that **MEANS THE SAME**. For example, "rich" and "wealthy" are synonyms.

RICH	WEALTHY
FAST	
SILLY	
CONQUER	
LOUD	
SMART	
LONG	
DIFFICULT	
THIEF	
TALK	
CUTE	

ANSWERS TO:
FILL IN the box with a
SYNONYM.

RICH	WEALTHY
FAST	QUICK
SILLY	FUNNY
CONQUER	VANQUISH
LOUD	NOISY
SMART	INTELLIGENT
LONG	LENGTHY
DIFFICULT	HARD
THIEF	ROBBER
TALK	SPEAK
CUTE	ADORABLE

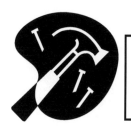

NAME the **ACTION** or **USE** of the **OBJECT**. For example, we tap a hammer.

HAMMER	TAP
FORK	
SHOVEL	
CLOCK	
TOWEL	
SPONGE	
SAW	
PIANO	
HORN	
CAR	
TV	

ANSWERS TO:
NAME the **ACTION** or
USE of the **OBJECT**.

HAMMER	TAP
FORK	EAT
SHOVEL	DIG
CLOCK	WIND, TELL TIME
TOWEL	DRY, WIPE
SPONGE	SQUEEZE, WIPE
SAW	SAW, CUT
PIANO	PLAY
HORN	BLOW
CAR	DRIVE
TV	WATCH

NAME the **ACTIVITY**, given the **TOOLS**. The first one is done for you.

jack, lug wrench, spare	change a flat tire
bucket, hose, sponge, soap, chamois cloth	
stationery, pen, envelope, stamp	
pretty paper, ribbon, tape, scissors, box	
seeds, trowel, watering can, soil, clay pot	
flashlight, costume, empty bag	
clothespins, clothesline, wet laundry	
bathing suit, blanket, towel, sunscreen	
bucket, shovel, wet sand or mud	
pumpkin, knife, spoon, candle	
soap, water, towel	

ANWERS TO:
NAME the **ACTIVITY,**
given the **TOOLS**.

jack, lug wrench, spare	change a flat tire
bucket, hose, sponge, soap, chamois cloth	wash a car
stationery, pen, envelope, stamp	write a letter
pretty paper, ribbon, tape, scissors, box	wrap a gift
seeds, trowel, watering can, soil, clay pot	plant a flower
flashlight, costume, empty bag	go trick-or-treating
clothespins, clothesline, wet laundry	hang clothes to dry
bathing suit, blanket, towel, sunscreen	go to the beach
bucket, shovel, wet sand or mud	make mud pies or sand castles
pumpkin, knife, spoon, candle	carve a jack-o-lantern
soap, water, towel	wash hands or face

> **NAME** the **OCCUPATION**,
> given the "tools of the trade."
> The first one is done for you.

ladder, hydrant, ax, extinguisher, hose	**firefighter**
stethoscope, thermometer, tongue depressor, scalpel	
hammer, nails, sander, tape measure, level	
wrench, copper pipe, soldering iron, snake	
pad, pencil, apron, tray, menu	
rod, reel, waders, bait, tackle	
brushes, drop cloths, tape, trays, rollers	
desks, books, pencils, white board, maps	
stage, microphone, lighting, music, speakers	
calculator, ledgers, pencil, computer	
stage, script, costume, audience, director	

ANSWERS TO:
NAME the OCCUPATION,
given the "tools of the trade."

ladder, hydrant, ax, extinguisher, hose	firefighter
stethoscope, thermometer, tongue depressor, scalpel	doctor
hammer, nails, sander, tape measure, level	carpenter
wrench, copper pipe, soldering iron, snake	plumber
pad, pencil, apron, tray, menu	waiter
rod, reel, waders, bait, tackle	angler, fishermen
brushes, drop cloths, tape, trays, rollers	painter
desks, books, pencils, white board, maps	teacher
stage, microphone, lighting, music, speakers	musician, singer
calculator, ledgers, pencil, computer	accountant
stage, script, costume, audience, director	actor

> **NAME** the **FOOD** or **BEVERAGE,** given the ingredients and tools. The first one is done for you.

broth, egg noodles, vegetables, salt, pepper, seasonings	vegetable soup
rice, ground beef & pork, spices, water, cabbage, tomatoes	
flour, baking powder, salt, sugar, milk, margarine	
milk, chocolate, marshmallows	
chocolate chips, nuts, condensed milk, butter, candy thermometer, pot	
yogurt, milk, fresh fruit, blender	
ice cream, sliced banana, whipped cream, topping, scoop	
ground round, spices, cheese, flipper, frying pan	
vodka, orange juice, ice	
bread crumbs, oil, flaked salmon, S & P, egg, onion, flour	

```
┌─────────────────────────────┐
│       ANSWERS TO:           │
│  NAME the FOOD or           │
│  BEVERAGE, given the        │
│   ingredients and tools     │
└─────────────────────────────┘
```

broth, egg noodles, vegetables, salt, pepper, seasonings	vegetable soup
rice, ground beef & pork, spices, water, cabbage, tomatoes	stuffed cabbage
flour, baking powder, salt, sugar, milk, margarine	cake
milk, chocolate, marshmallows	hot chocolate
chocolate chips, nuts, condensed milk, butter, candy thermometer, pot	fudge
yogurt, milk, fresh fruit, blender	smoothie
ice cream, sliced banana, whipped cream, topping, scoop	banana split
ground round, spices, cheese, flipper, frying pan	cheeseburger
vodka, orange juice, ice	screwdriver
bread crumbs, oil, flaked salmon, S & P, egg, onion, flour	salmon patties

NAME the FAMOUS LOCATION.

1. The waterfalls that straddle the border between the US and Canada are _____

2. A famous cathedral in Paris, France is _____

3. The capital of Poland is _____

4. The most famous intersection in NY City is _____

5. The Italian city known for its many small islands separated by canals and linked by bridges is _____

6. The US city known for some of the largest hotels, resorts and casinos in the world is _____

7. The only one of the seven great wonders of the ancient world that is still standing is the Great _____

8. A famous site in England, composed of a circular setting of large standing stones is_____

9. A monument in Boston, to commemorate a battle in the American Revolutionary War, is _____

10. The large, gothic church in London, where weddings, coronations and funerals of royalty take place is

_____

> ## ANSWERS TO:
> ## NAME the FAMOUS LOCATION.

1. The waterfalls that straddle the border between the US and Canada are ___Niagara Falls___

2. A famous cathedral in Paris, France is ___Notre Dame___

3. The capital of Poland is ___Warsaw___

4. The famous intersection in NY City is ___Times Square___

5. The Italian city known for its many small islands separated by canals and linked by bridges is ___Venice___

6. The US city known for some of the largest hotels, resorts and casinos in the world is ___Las Vegas___

7. The only one of the seven great wonders of the ancient world that is still standing is the Great ___Pyramid___

8. A famous site in England, composed of a circular setting of large standing stones is___Stonehenge___

9. A monument in Boston, to commemorate a battle in the American Revolutionary War, is ___Bunker Hill___

10. The large, gothic church in London, where weddings, coronations and funerals of royalty take place is ___Westminster Cathedral___

FILL IN the **BLANK** to
IDENTIFY a **PERSON**.
Note: There may be more
than one correct answer.

1. A person who studies the past by excavating and uncovering old relics is an _____

2. The first woman to win a Nobel Prize for her pioneering research on radioactivity was _____

3. A renowned child-prodigy pianist and composer who grew up in Poland was _____

4. The person who rides horses in races as a profession is called a _____

5. The ruler in a monarchy is typically a _____

6. A person very new to a field or activity is a _____

7. A person who lacks the skill of a professional is called an _____

8. One group of tall, women warriors were called

_____

9. A singer whose voice range lies between soprano and tenor is an _____

10. A person with fair hair and skin and usually light eyes is a _____

> ## ANSWERS TO:
> ## FILL IN the BLANK to
> ## IDENTIFY a PERSON.

1. A person who studies the past by excavating and uncovering old relics is an ___archeologist___

2. The first woman to win a Nobel Prize for her pioneering research on radioactivity was ___Marie Curie___

3. A renowned child-prodigy pianist and composer who grew up in Poland was ___Chopin___

4. The person who rides horses in races as a profession is called a ___jockey___

5. The ruler in a monarchy is typically a ___king or queen___

6. A person very new to a field or activity is a ___novice___

7. A person who lacks the skill of a professional is called an ___amateur___

8. One group of tall, women warriors were called ___Amazons___

9. A singer whose voice range lies between soprano and tenor is an ___alto___

10. A person with fair hair and skin and usually light eyes is a ___blonde___

???

FILL IN the BLANK to IDENTIFY an OBJECT. Note: There may be more than one correct answer.

1. The flower of a plant is called its _____

2. The headpiece worn by a king or queen is a _____

3. A type of sweater without sleeves is a _____

4. A unit of measure equal to 3 feet is a _____

5. A nine-branched candelabrum used in celebration of Hanukkah is a _____

6. A card with space on one side for an address and stamp and space on the other side for a short message is a

   _____

7. An inclined surface to connect different levels, especially helpful to people in wheelchairs, is a _____

8. Dried grapes often found in cereal are _____

9. The equipment used in fishing is called _____

10. A small amount of money given to someone for their service is called a _____

ANSWERS TO:
FILL IN the BLANK to
IDENTIFY an OBJECT.

1. The flower of a plant is called its __blossom__

2. The headpiece worn by a king or queen is a __crown__

3. A type of sweater without sleeves is a __vest__

4. A unit of measure equal to 3 feet is a __yard__

5. A nine-branched candelabrum used in celebration of Hanukkah is a __menorah__

6. A card with space on one side for an address and stamp and space on the other side for a short message is a __post card__

7. An inclined surface to connect different levels, especially helpful to people in wheelchairs, is a __ramp__

8. Dried grapes often found in cereal are __raisins__

9. The equipment used in fishing is called __tackle__

10. A small amount of money given to someone for their service is called a __tip__

???

FILL IN the **BLANK** to **IDENTIFY** a **PLACE**. Note: There may be more than one correct answer.

1. The pointed summit of a mountain is its _____

2. Ground on which grass or other vegetation grows for grazing animals is called a _____

3. An exhibition where skills like riding broncos or roping calves are displayed is a _____

4. The center of colonial towns was often called the town _____

5. A building or room to exhibit artists' work is a _____

6. A large amphitheatre for public events, including an ancient one where gladiators fought, is a _____

7. Theatre actors typically perform on a _____

8. If you want a safe place to store cash and jewels, you might choose a safety deposit _____

9. A place were minerals are extracted from the earth is a _____

10. Wild animals at the zoo are restricted in _____

> ## <u>ANSWERS TO:</u>
> ### FILL IN the BLANK to
> ### IDENTIFY a <u>PLACE</u>.

1. The pointed summit of a mountain is its __peak__

2. Ground on which grass or other vegetation grows for grazing animals is called a ___pasture___

3. An exhibition where skills like riding broncos or roping calves are displayed is a ___rodeo___

4. The center of colonial towns was often called the town ___green or square___

5. A building or room to exhibit artists' work is a <u>gallery</u>

6. A large amphitheatre for public events, including an ancient one where gladiators fought, is a <u>coliseum</u>

7. Theatre actors typically perform on a <u>stage</u>

8. If you want a safe place to store cash and jewels, you might choose a safety deposit <u>box</u>

9. A place were minerals are extracted from the earth is a <u>mine</u>

10. Wild animals at the zoo are restricted in <u>cages</u>

???

> Think about **TIME OR EVENTS** and **FILL IN** the **BLANK**. Note: There may be more than one correct answer.

1. Restaurants offer drinks at half price at a time in early evening called _____

2. Universities offer incoming freshmen a time to become acquainted during _____

3. Houses on the market are often shown to prospective buyers at an event called an _____

4. The first showing of a movie is its _____

5. People who are moving often try to sell possessions at a

   _____

6. The major dance for high school students during their junior and senior years is the _____

7. The holiday associated with dressing in costumes is

   _____

8. Flowers first bloom in the season of _____

9. The "Day of Reckoning" is a term used to describe the Christian belief in _____

10. According to the Old Testament, Noah built an ark to prepare for the great _____

> ## ANSWERS TO:
> Think about **TIME OR EVENTS** and **FILL IN** the **BLANK**.

1. Restaurants offer drinks at half price at a time in early evening called ____happy hour____

2. Universities offer incoming freshmen a time to become acquainted during ____orientation____

3. Houses on the market are often shown to prospective buyers at an event called an ___open house___

4. The first showing of a movie is its __premier__

5. People who are moving often try to sell possessions at a ____garage sale or tag sale or yard sale____

6. The major dance for high school students during their junior and senior years is the ____prom____

7. The holiday associated with dressing in costumes is ____Halloween____

8. Flowers first bloom in the season of ___spring___

9. The "Day of Reckoning" is a term used to describe the Christian belief in __Judgment Day or an afterlife__

10. According to the Old Testament, Noah built an ark to prepare for the great ___flood___

??? THINK ABOUT <u>REASONS</u> WE DO THINGS</u> and FILL IN the BLANK. Note: There may be more than one correct answer.

1. We carry a jack in the trunk to fix a _____

2. To prevent flooding in your basement, you might install a _____

3. I might keep a bucket of sand in my trunk during winter months in case of _____

4. Objects fall to the ground because of _____

5. A nurse uses a thermometer to tell whether a patient has a _____

6. To quickly defrost meat, you might place it in the

   _____

7. Doctors often prescribe antibiotics to cure an

   _____

8. We use potholders in the kitchen to prevent _____

9. To fill the tub with water, you turn on the _____

10. To empty the tub, you open the _____

```
┌─────────────────────────────────┐
│          ANSWERS TO:            │
│    THINK ABOUT REASONS          │
│   WE DO THINGS and FILL IN      │
│         the BLANK.              │
└─────────────────────────────────┘
```

1. We carry a jack in the trunk to fix a ___flat tire___

2. To prevent flooding in your basement, you might install a ___sump pump___

3. I might keep a bucket of sand in my trunk during winter months in case of ___ice or snow___

4. Objects fall to the ground because of ___gravity___

5. A nurse uses a thermometer to tell whether a patient has a ___temperature___

6. To quickly defrost meat, you might place it in the ___microwave___

7. Doctors often prescribe antibiotics to cure an ___infection___

8. We use potholders in the kitchen to prevent ___burns___

9. To fill the tub with water, you turn on the ___faucet___

10. To empty the tub, you open the ___drain___

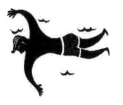

> **CIRCLE** the **SUMMER OLYMPIC SPORTS** that appear on the 3 lists below. You should find 15 sports all together. Good luck!

List 1	List 2	List 3
swimming	driving	sailing
luge	reading	skiing
archery	snowboarding	rowing
diving	gymnastics	volleyball
badminton	fencing	arm wrestling
sewing	field hockey	knitting
pruning	sledding	ice hockey
riding	hiking	cooking
canoeing	water polo	tennis
cycling	bobsleigh	shooting
curling	baking	ski jumping

ANSWERS TO
CIRCLE 15 <u>SUMMER</u>
<u>OLYMPIC SPORTS</u>.

<u>List 1</u>	<u>List 2</u>	<u>List 3</u>
swimming		sailing
archery		rowing
diving	gymnastics	volleyball
badminton	fencing	
	field hockey	
canoeing	water polo	tennis
cycling		shooting

NAME 10 TOPPINGS on
a **PIZZA**. HINT: Think of
meats and vegetables.

1. _____

2. _____

3. _____

4. _____

5. _____

6. _____

7. _____

8. _____

9. _____

10. _____

ANSWERS TO:
NAME 10 TOPPINGS on
a **PIZZA**.

---

1.   cheese

2.   pepperoni

3.   sausage

4.   hamburger

5.   anchovies

6.   mushrooms

7.   tomatoes

8.   broccoli

9.   spinach

10. onions

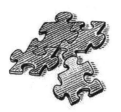

> **READ** the **ITEMS**; then **NAME** the **CATEGORY**. For example, "dog, cat, bird, goldfish and hamster" go together because they belong to the category of "pets."

ITEMS	CATEGORY
dog, cat, bird, goldfish, hamster	pets
sneakers, shoes, boots, slippers, socks	
pants, slacks, jeans, trousers, tights	
Ice skating, skiing, sledding, snowboarding	
Snicker's, Almond Joy, Mounds, Milky Way	
ringmaster, clowns, elephants, acrobats	
engine, trunk, chassis, tires, steering wheel	
candle, lamp, lantern, chandelier, flashlight	
oxygen, carbon, iron, copper, gold	
Cancer, Virgo, Libra, Taurus, Capricorn	

```
┌─────────────────────────────────┐
│      ANSWERS TO:                │
│   READ the ITEMS; then          │
│   NAME the CATEGORY.            │
└─────────────────────────────────┘
```

ITEMS	CATEGORY
dog, cat, bird, goldfish, hamster	pets
sneakers, shoes, boots, slippers, socks	footwear
pants, slacks, jeans, trousers, tights	clothing worn on our legs
Ice skating, skiing, sledding, snowboarding	winter sports
Snicker's, Almond Joy, Mounds, Milky Way	chocolate bars
ringmaster, clowns, elephants, acrobats	things in a circus
engine, trunk, chassis, tires, steering wheel	parts of a car
candle, lamp, lantern, chandelier, flashlight	sources of light
oxygen, carbon, iron, copper, gold	elements
Cancer, Virgo, Libra, Taurus, Capricorn	astrological signs

FOCUS on the
SUPERMARKET and
FILL IN the **BLANK**.

1. The spaces between rows of shelves are **a**_____

2. The department that sells lunch meat and cheese is the **d**_____

3. The supervisor of the store and each department is called the **m**_____

4. Shoppers can check out without the help of a cashier at the **s**_____

5. Many shoppers choose to pay a cashier who operates the **c**_____

6. The one bad person **a**_____

7. Customers place their items in a shopping **c**_____

8. Shoppers get discounts by using manufacturers' or store **c**_____

9. People might call a wonderful invention, "the greatest thing since sliced **b**_____"

10. Unscramble these words (related to a supermarket):

    D U C P O R E   _____

    Z E R E F R E   _____

    Y C N A D   _____

    G A M Z N E I A   _____

    R Y A B E K   _____

> ## ANSWERS TO:
> ### FOCUS on the
> ## SUPERMARKET.

1. The spaces between rows of shelves are <u>aisles</u>

2. The department that sells lunch meat and cheese is the <u>delicatessen</u>

3. The supervisor of the store and each department is called the <u>manager</u>

4. Shoppers can check out without the help of a cashier at the <u>self-service lane</u>

5. Many shoppers choose to pay a cashier who operates the <u>cash register</u>

6. The bad person in a group is called the "rotten <u>apple</u>"

7. Customers place their items in a shopping <u>cart</u>

8. Shoppers get discounts by using manufacturers' or store <u>coupons</u>

9. People might call a wonderful invention, "the greatest thing since sliced <u>bread</u>   "

10. Unscramble these words (related to a supermarket):

    D U C P O R E   <u>produce</u>

    Z E R E F R E   <u>freezer</u>

    Y C N A D   <u>candy</u>

    G A M Z N E I A   <u>magazine</u>

    R Y A B E K   <u>bakery</u>

 **FILL IN** the **BOX** with the **WORD THAT DOESN'T BELONG**. For example, "dog, cat, goldfish and hamster" are all pets; "fork" is NOT a pet—it doesn't belong in the group.

ITEMS	DOESN'T BELONG
dog, cat, fork, goldfish, hamster	fork
Parmesan, Swiss, Cheddar, Bacon, American	
knife, scissors, staple, saw, ax	
square, diamond, circle, rectangle, trapezoid	
touch, see, kick, hear, smell	
puppy, kitty, horse, chick, duckling	
crayon, marker, ruler, pencil, pen	
plane, helicopter, blimp, trolley, jet	
nickel, dime, peso, dollar, quarter	
bottle, diaper, bib, bra, blanket	

ANSWERS TO:
FILL IN the BOX with the WORD
THAT DOESN'T BELONG

ITEMS	DOESN'T BELONG
dog, cat, fork, goldfish, hamster	fork
Parmesan, Swiss, Cheddar, Bacon, American	Bacon
knife, scissors, staple, saw, ax	staple
square, diamond, circle, rectangle, trapezoid	circle
touch, see, kick, hear, smell	kick
puppy, kitty, horse, chick, duckling	horse
crayon, marker, ruler, pencil, pen	ruler
plane, helicopter, blimp, trolley, jet	trolley
nickel, dime, peso, dollar, quarter	peso
bottle, diaper, bib, bra, blanket	bra

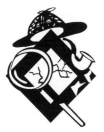

Use the clues to help you
NAME the **WORD**.

Clue	Answer
1. A flightless bird, with a long neck and long, fast legs, is an	O _ _ _ _ _ _
2. An exaggerated and/or false legend passed down to youth is called an "old wife's	T _ _ _
3. Pirates sometimes forced their captives to walk the	P _ _ _ _
4. An appliance with blades that spin to cool the air is a	F _ _
5. A body of land surrounded by water is an	I _ _ _ _ _
6. Some manufacturers offer to replace their items if still under	W _ _ _ _ _ _ _
7. The official count of the population, taken every ten years, is the	C _ _ _ _ _
8. Police officers may stop speeders and give them a	T _ _ _ _ _
9. Trains that carry cargo rather than passengers are this type of train	F _ _ _ _ _ _

> ## <u>ANSWERS TO:</u>
> Use the clues to help you
> **NAME** the **<u>WORD</u>**.

1. A flightless bird, with a long neck and long, fast legs, is an	**ostrich**
2. An exaggerated and/or false legend passed down to youth is called an "old wife's	**tale**
3. Pirates sometimes forced their captives to walk the	**plank**
4. An appliance with blades that spin to cool the air is a	**fan**
5. A body of land surrounded by water is an	**island**
6. Some manufacturers offer to replace their items if still under	**warranty**
7. The official count of the population, taken every ten years, is the	**census**
8. Police officers may stop speeders and give them a	**ticket**
9. Trains that carry cargo rather than passengers are this type of train	**freight**

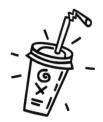

UNSCRAMBLE the
LETTERS to make a word.
HINT: All of the words are
BEVERAGES. The first one is
done for you.

E E B R	B E E R
R W T A E	W _ _ _ _
M O L E N D E A	L _ _ _ _ _ _ _
T Z S E R L E	S _ _ _ _ _ _
U C I E J	J _ _ _ _
C U N P H	P _ _ _ _
S D O A	S _ _ _
N E W I	W _ _ _
F F E O C E	C _ _ _ _ _
I M K L	M _ _ _

ANSWERS TO:
UNSCRAMBLE the
LETTERS to make a word.

E E B R   **BEER**

R WT A E   **WATER**

M O L E N D E A **LEMONADE**

T Z S E R L E   **SELTZER**

U C I E J   **JUICE**

C U N P H   **PUNCH**

S D O A   **SODA**

N E W I   **WINE**

F F E O C E   **COFFEE**

I M K L   **MILK**

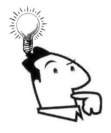

PICTURE the DESCRIPTION;
then FILL IN the BLANK.

1. I am a fairytale character, a woman dressed in black who flies on a broomstick. I am a _____

2. I am a forest animal known to carry tics that can cause Lyme disease. I am a _____

3. I am a round adornment hung on the front door of homes, decorated with leaves, flowers and a bow. I am a _____

4. I am a character made from three large snowballs, a corncob pipe and eyes of coal. I am a _____

5. I am a shiny silver paper, used in cooking and storing food. I am _____

6. I am a fast ride at an amusement park, with cars hooked together on loops of track. I am a _____

7. I am another amusement park ride, with gondolas on a rotating upright wheel. I am a _____

8. I am elasticized straps used to hold up trousers. I am

_____

9. I am folded flaps of cloth on the front of a jacket or coat. I am _____

10. I am a packaging item, made of paper or thin cardboard, used to mail a letter or card. I am an

_____

ANSWERS TO:
PICTURE the DESCRIPTION.

1. I am a fairytale character, a woman dressed in black who flies on a broomstick. I am a __witch__

2. I am a forest animal known to carry tics that can cause Lyme disease. I am a __deer__

3. I am a round adornment hung on the front door of homes, decorated with leaves, flowers and a bow. I am a __wreath__

4. I am a character made from three large snowballs, a corncob pipe and eyes of coal. I am a __snowman__

5. I am a shiny silver paper, used in cooking and storing food. I am __tin foil__

6. I am a fast ride at an amusement park, with cars hooked together on loops of track. I am a __roller coaster__

7. I am another amusement park ride, with gondolas on a rotating upright wheel. I am a __ferris wheel__

8. I am elasticized straps used to hold up trousers. I am __suspenders__

9. I am folded flaps of cloth on the front of a jacket or coat. I am __lapels__

10. I am a packaging item, made of paper or thin cardboard, used to mail a letter or card. I am an __envelope__

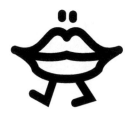

COMPLETE the COMMON SAYING.

1. A person who looks sick might be described as looking, "a little green around the _____"

2. A couple who get along perfectly are said to have a "match made in _____"

3. When people eat a meal and then leave quickly, they "eat and _____"

4. A man who gets in trouble with his wife is "in the _____"

5. Someone who spends most of his time alone and has few friends is called "a lone _____"

6. You might advise someone to watch very carefully by saying, "keep your eyes _____"

7. An important person or leader in business is often called "the big _____"

8. When a professional opens their own business, we say that they "hang out their own _____"

9. A perfectly fitting dress might be described as "fitting like a _____"

10. When we accomplished two goals with one action, we "kill two birds with one _____"

<u>ANSWERS TO</u>:
COMPLETE the **<u>COMMON</u>**
<u>SAYING</u>.

1. A person who looks sick might be described as looking, "a little green around the ___gills___ "

2. A couple who get along perfectly are said to have a "match made in ___heaven___ "

3. When people eat a meal and then leave quickly, they "eat and___run___ "

4. A man who gets in trouble with his wife is "in the ___dog house___ "

5. Someone who spends most of his time alone and has few friends is called "a lone___wolf___ "

6. You might advise someone to watch very carefully by saying, "keep your eyes ___peeled___ "

7. An important person or leader in business is often called "the big ___cheese___ "

8. When a professional opens their own business, we say that they "hang out their own ___shingle___ "

9. A perfectly fitting dress might be described as "fitting like a___glove___ "

10. When we accomplished two goals with one action, we "kill two birds with one ___stone___ "

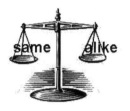

FILL IN the box with a **SYNONYM,** a word that **MEANS THE SAME**. For example, "rich" and "wealthy" are synonyms.

RICH	**WEALTHY**
EASY	
STRAINER	
CAR	
BUCKET	
AGREE	
DEARTH	
SOLID	
LAUNCH	
PLIABLE	
METAMORPHOSIS	

ANSWERS TO:
FILL IN the box with a
SYNONYM.

RICH	WEALTHY
EASY	SIMPLE
STRAINER	COLANDER
CAR	AUTOMOBILE
BUCKET	PAIL
AGREE	CONCUR
DEARTH	SHORTAGE
SOLID	FIRM
LAUNCH	START
PLIABLE	FLEXIBLE
METAMORPHOSIS	CHANGE

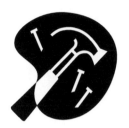

NAME the **ACTION** or
USE of the **OBJECT**. For
example, we tap a hammer.

HAMMER	TAP
WHISTLE	
DRUMS	
SCISSORS	
CRAYON	
COLANDER	
DVD	
CD	
BELL	
RULER	
RADIO	

ANSWERS TO:
NAME the **ACTION** or
USE of the **OBJECT**.

HAMMER	TAP
WHISTLE	BLOW
DRUMS	BEAT
SCISSORS	CUT
CRAYON	COLOR
COLANDER	STRAIN
DVD	WATCH
CD	LISTEN TO
BELL	RING
RULER	MEASURE
RADIO	LISTEN TO

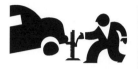 NAME the **ACTIVITY**, given the **TOOLS**. The first one is done for you.

jack, lug wrench, spare	change a flat tire
list, wallet, cart, coupons, empty soda bottles/cans	
map or GPS, luggage, motel reservations, credit card	
comb, water, shampoo, sharp scissors, mirror, towel	
cuticle clippers, polish remover, polish, file	
mattress pad, pillow cases, sheets, pillows, blankets	
tent, sleeping bags, tarp, hatchet, matches	
pastry bag, tips, icing, spoon, knife, cake	
large sharp knife, cutting board, platter, big fork, apron	
tickets, popcorn, drink	
bowl, flakes, milk, sugar, tablespoon, teaspoon	

> ## ANSWERS TO:
> ## NAME the ACTIVITY,
> ### given the TOOLS.

jack, lug wrench, spare	change a flat tire
list, wallet, cart, coupons, empty soda bottles/cans	grocery shop
map or GPS, luggage, motel reservations, credit card	vacation
comb, water, shampoo, sharp scissors, mirror, towel	cut hair
cuticle clippers, polish remover, polish, file	manicure
mattress pad, pillow cases, sheets, pillows, blankets	change a bed
tent, sleeping bags, tarp, hatchet, matches	camp
pastry bag, tips, icing, spoon, knife, cake	decorate a cake
large sharp knife, cutting board, platter, big fork, apron	carve a roast
tickets, popcorn, drink	go to a movie
bowl, flakes, milk, sugar, tablespoon, teaspoon	breakfast

> # NAME the __OCCUPATION,__
> given the "tools of the trade."
> The first one is done for you.

ladder, hydrant, ax, extinguisher, hose	**firefighter**
vision charts, dilating drops, lens holders	
weights, exercise bolsters, balls and tubing	
deep fryer, griddle, spoon, flipper, measuring spoons/cups	
cement, trowel, level, plumb bob, bricks	
iridescent vest or jacket, hand-held stop sign	
utility knives, staple gun, glue gun, stretchers	
barcode scanner, cash register, receipts, credit card scanner	
standardized tests, computer, __Diagnostic and Statistical Manual of Mental Disorders__	
books, barcode scanners, microfiche readers, computer	
red suit, white beard	

ANSWERS TO:
NAME the **OCCUPATION**,
given the "tools of the trade."

ladder, hydrant, ax, extinguisher, hose	firefighter
vision charts, dilating drops, lens holders	eye doctor
weights, exercise bolsters, balls and tubing	physical therapist
deep fryer, griddle, spoon, flipper, measuring spoons/cups	short order cook
cement, trowel, level, plumb bob, bricks	mason
iridescent vest or jacket, hand-held stop sign	crossing guard
utility knives, staple gun, glue gun, stretchers	carpet layer
barcode scanner, cash register, receipts, credit card scanner	cashier
standardized tests, computer, Diagnostic and Statistical Manual of Mental Disorders	psychologist
books, barcode scanners, microfiche readers, computer	librarian
red suit, white beard	Santa

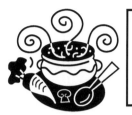

NAME the **FOOD** or **BEVERAGE,** given the ingredients and tools. The first one is done for you.

broth, egg noodles, vegetables, salt, pepper, seasonings	vegetable soup
tuna fish, mayo, celery, pepper, bread	
crust, mozzarella, tomato sauce, pepperoni, Italian seasoning	
ground beef, kidney beans, black beans, tomatoes, green pepper, chili powder, cayenne	
open flame, chocolate bar, marshmallows, graham crackers	
hard-boiled eggs, salt & pepper, paprika, salad dressing	
milk, sugar, cornstarch, vanilla, salt, butter, pot	
ground beef, onion, garlic, refried beans, olives, taco sauce, tortillas, cheese	
vodka, tomato juice, Worcestershire sauce	
buns, franks, mustard, relish, sauerkraut	

> **ANWERS TO:**
> **NAME** the **FOOD** or
> **BEVERAGE,** given the
> ingredients and tools.

broth, egg noodles, vegetables, salt, pepper, seasonings	vegetable soup
tuna fish, mayo, celery, pepper, bread	tuna fish sandwich
crust, mozzarella, tomato sauce, pepperoni, Italian seasoning	pizza
ground beef, kidney beans, black beans, tomatoes, green pepper, chili powder, cayenne	chili
open flame, chocolate bar, marshmallows, graham crackers	s'mores
hard-boiled eggs, salt & pepper, paprika, salad dressing	deviled eggs
milk, sugar, cornstarch, vanilla, salt, butter, pot	pudding
ground beef, onion, garlic, refried beans, olives, taco sauce, tortillas, cheese	enchiladas
vodka, tomato juice, Worcestershire sauce	Bloody Mary
buns, franks, mustard, relish, sauerkraut	hot dogs

NAME the FAMOUS LOCATION.

1. The famous waterway between the Atlantic and Pacific Oceans is the _____

2. A national memorial that features sculptures of the heads of four US presidents is _____

3. The geographic location that marks the separation of the watersheds of the Pacific Ocean from those of the Atlantic and Arctic Oceans is the_____

4. The extensive fortification built to protect China's border is the _____

5. The tallest structure in Paris and one of the most visited monuments in the word is the _____

6. The famous location of Russia's government is the

    _____

7. The famous 1939-1940 exposition held in Flushing Meadows, New York with an opening slogan, "Dawn of a New Day," was the _____

8. The result of the Colorado River and its tributaries cutting through layers of rock for billions of years is the natural wonder called the _____

ANSWERS TO:
NAME the FAMOUS LOCATION.

1. The famous waterway between the Atlantic and Pacific Oceans is the __Panama Canal__

2. A national memorial that features sculptures of the heads of four US presidents is __Mount Rushmore__

3. The geographic location that marks the separation of the watersheds of the Pacific Ocean from those of the Atlantic and Arctic Oceans is the __Continental Divide__

4. The extensive fortification built to protect China's border is the __Great Wall__

5. The tallest structure in Paris and one of the most visited monuments in the word is the __Eiffel Tower__

6. The famous location of Russia's government is the

   __Kremlin__

7. The famous 1939-1940 exposition held in Flushing Meadows, New York with an opening slogan, "Dawn of a New Day," was the __World's Fair__

8. The result of the Colorado River and its tributaries cutting through layers of rock for billions of years is the natural wonder called the __Grand Canyon__

???

> **FILL IN** the **BLANK** to **IDENTIFY** a **PERSON**.
> Note: There may be more than one correct answer.

1. People who bring their faith to distant lands are called

   _____

2. A leader who assumes abusive powers, sometimes without election or civil liberties, is a _____

3. A person who sells old collectibles is an antique_____

4. People who help clients buy and sell homes are called real estate _____

5. The head of the Police Department typically has the title of _____

6. The second in command in United States government is the _____

7. A person who gets secret information without permission is a secret agent or _____

8. The person in charge of all things related to a kitchen is the _____

9. The person responsible for training and developing an athletic team is the _____

10. A homeless, unemployed person is a _____

ANSWERS TO:
FILL IN the **BLANK** to
IDENTIFY a **PERSON**.

---

1. People who bring their faith to distant lands are called
   missionaries

2. A leader who assumes abusive powers, sometimes
   without election or civil liberties, is a __dictator__

3. A person who sells old collectibles is an antique
   dealer

4. People who help clients buy and sell homes are called
   real estate __agents or brokers__

5. The head of the Police Department typically has the
   title of ____Chief

6. The second in command in United States government is
   the ____Vice President

7. A person who gets secret information without
   permission is a secret agent or ____spy

8. The person in charge of all things related to a kitchen is
   the ____chef

9. The person responsible for training and developing an
   athletic team is the ____coach

10. A homeless, unemployed person is a ____vagrant

FILL IN the BLANK to
IDENTIFY an OBJECT.
Note: There may be more
than one correct answer.

1. The attachment at the end of a hose is the _____

2. A tool used to remove splinters is a pair of _____

3. A leaky faucet may be fixed by replacing a _____

4. Children chase one another in an age-old game called

   _____

5. The yard tool used to collect fallen leaves is a _____

6. An outdoor wooden seat for several people in a park is

   a _____

7. A textile floor covering is a _____

8. Children go trick-or-treating in hope of getting lots of

   _____

9. The part of an automobile that holds gasoline is the

   _____

10. The hard candy that comes on a stick is a_____

> ## ANSWERS TO:
> ### FILL IN the BLANK to IDENTIFY an OBJECT.

1. The attachment at the end of a hose is the ___nozzle___

2. A tool used to remove splinters is a pair of tweezers____

3. A leaky faucet may be fixed by replacing a _washer____

4. Children chase one another in an age-old game called _____tag_____

5. The yard tool used to collect fallen leaves is a _rake___

6. An outdoor wooden seat for several people in a park is a _____bench_____

7. A textile floor covering is a ____rug or carpet_____

8. Children go trick-or-treating in hope of getting lots of _____candy_____

9. The part of an automobile that holds gasoline is the _____gas tank_____

10. The hard candy that comes on a stick is a_lollipop____

???

FILL IN the **BLANK** to **IDENTIFY** a **PLACE**. Note: There may be more than one correct answer.

1. To reach the tenth floor, people take the _____

2. Dalmatians, ladders and sirens are associated with a

   _____

3. During remodeling, old building materials are discarded

   in a _____

4. The fancy entranceway to a house is the _____

5. Ships are guided into harbor by a tall, circular building

   with a beacon, known as a _____

6. Expansive, expensive homes are called _____

7. The building that houses local government is the

   _____

8. Very tall buildings in metropolitan areas are sometimes

   called _____

9. The tall tower on a church or building is the_____

10. The underground room in medieval castles, where

    prisoners were held, was the _____

> ### ANSWERS TO:
> ### FILL IN the BLANK to
> ### IDENTIFY a PLACE.

1. To reach the tenth floor, people take the __elevator__

2. Dalmatians, ladders and sirens are associated with a __fire station__

3. During remodeling, old building materials are discarded in a __dumpster__

4. The fancy entranceway to a house is the __foyer__

5. Ships are guided into harbor by a tall, circular building with a beacon, known as a __lighthouse__

6. Expansive, expensive homes are called __mansions__

7. The building that houses local government is the __town or city hall__

8. Very tall buildings in metropolitan areas are sometimes called __skyscrapers__

9. The tall tower on a church or building is the __spire or steeple__

10. The underground room in medieval castles, where prisoners were held, was the __dungeon__

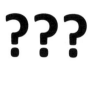

Think about **TIME OR EVENTS** and **FILL IN** the **BLANK.** Note: There may be more than one correct answer.

1. As a symbol of respect, the flag is flown at _____

2. "Taps" is a song played by the military at funerals or at

_____

3. TV commercials are played during _____

4. On New Years Day, people make promises called

_____

5. Every six months, people often make an appointment for a teeth-cleaning at the _____

6. Holidays associated with parades are Memorial Day and the _____

7. Following an auto accident, victims are taken by ambulance to a _____

8. When performers return to the stage to sing yet another song, they are giving an _____

9. Before the main meal is served, guests often enjoy

a variety of _____

10. People typically remember more dreams during a period of sleep called _____

ANSWERS TO:
Think about **TIME OR EVENTS** and **FILL IN** the **BLANK.**

---

1. As a symbol of respect, the flag is flown at <u>half mast</u>

2. "Taps" is a song played by the military at funerals or at <u>dusk</u>

3. TV commercials are played during <u>intermissions</u>

4. On New Years Day, people make promises called <u>resolutions</u>

5. Every six months, people often make an appointment for a teeth-cleaning at the <u>dentist</u>

6. Holidays associated with parades are Memorial Day and the <u>Fourth of July</u>

7. Following an auto accident, victims are taken by ambulance to a <u>hospital</u>

8. When performers return to the stage to sing yet another song, they are giving an <u>encore</u>

9. Before the main meal is served, guests often enjoy a variety of <u>appetizers</u>

10. People typically remember more dreams during a period of sleep called <u>REM</u>

THINK ABOUT REASONS WE DO THINGS and **FILL IN** the **BLANK**. Note: There may be more than one correct answer.

1. In order to ensure delivery, letters must have the correct _____

2. When our doctor wants to check the rate and regularity of our heartbeats, he orders an _____

3. We turn the clocks back on the first weekend of November to return to _____

4. The amount of postage needed on a package is determined by its destination and _____

5. School districts expecting weather conditions to improve by mid-morning, may announce a_____

6. Long-lasting, dangerous road conditions may cause school districts to announce a _____

7. Elderly folks who are home alone may feel more secure if they wear a safety alarm called a _____

8. A car that runs out of gas, when the tank is supposed to be half full, may have a problem with the gas _____

9. You may need to sharpen scissors or a knife when they seem to be very _____

10. In order to keep our place in a novel we are reading, we might insert a _____

> # ANSWERS TO:
> # THINK ABOUT REASONS
> # WE DO THINGS and FILL IN
> # the BLANK.

1. In order to ensure delivery, letters must have the correct ___postage or address___

2. When our doctor wants to check the rate and regularity of our heartbeats, he orders an ___EKG___

3. We turn the clocks back on the first weekend of November to return to ___Eastern Standard Time___

4. The amount of postage needed on a package is determined by its destination and ___weight___

5. School districts expecting weather conditions to improve by mid-morning, may announce a ___delayed opening___

6. Long-lasting, dangerous road conditions may cause school districts to announce a ___cancellation___

7. Elderly folks who are home alone may feel more secure if they wear a safety alarm called a ___lifeline___

8. A car that runs out of gas, when the tank is supposed to be half full, may have a problem with the gas ___gauge___

9. You may need to sharpen scissors or a knife when they seem to be very ___dull___

10. In order to keep our place in a novel we are reading, we might insert a ___bookmark___

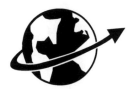

> **CIRCLE** the **NAMES OF COUNTRIES** that appear on the 3 lists below. You should find 15 countries all together. Good luck!

List 1	List 2	List 3
Asia	Rome	Syria
United States	Quebec	California
Africa	Mexico	Atlanta
New Zealand	Pacific	Indiana
Nova Scotia	Ireland	Russia
Arctic	Atlantic	India
Spain	London	Ghana
Iran	China	Moscow
Paris	Lisbon	Canada
Argentina	Cairo	Japan
Mississippi	Indonesia	Ohio

**ANSWERS TO:
CIRCLE the NAMES OF
15 COUNTRIES**

List 1	List 2	List 3
		Syria
United States		
	Mexico	
New Zealand		
	Ireland	Russia
		India
Spain		Ghana
Iran	China	
		Canada
Argentina		Japan
	Indonesia	

NAME 10 <u>COLLEGE MAJORS</u>. HINT: Think of school subjects and professional occupations.

1. _____

2. _____

3. _____

4. _____

5. _____

6. _____

7. _____

8. _____

9. _____

10. _____

ANSWERS TO:
NAME 10 <u>COLLEGE</u>
<u>MAJORS</u>.

1.   history
2.   English
3.   biology
4.   nursing
5.   architecture
6.   math
7.   education
8.   journalism
9.   art
10. music

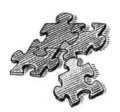

READ the ITEMS, then NAME the CATEGORY. For example, "dog, cat, bird, goldfish and hamster" go together because they belong to the category of "pets."

ITEMS	CATEGORY
dog, cat, bird, goldfish, hamster	pets
stove, sink, fridge, table, cabinets	
bed, dresser, closet, rug, TV	
tent, sleeping bag, gas stove, firewood	
screwdriver, hammer, wrench, pliers, saw	
ring, bracelet, necklace, earrings	
rod, reel, lures, bait, net	
needle, thread, pins, thimble, pattern	
bottle, diaper, crib, formula, rattle	
barn, silo, livestock, crops, tractor	

ANSWERS TO: NAME the CATEGORY.

ITEMS	CATEGORY
dog, cat, bird, goldfish, hamster	pets
stove, sink, fridge, table, cabinets	kitchen items
bed, dresser, closet, rug, TV	bedroom items
tent, sleeping bag, gas stove, firewood	camping items
screwdriver, hammer, wrench, pliers, saw	building tools
ring, bracelet, necklace, earrings	jewelry
rod, reel, lures, bait, net	fishing gear
needle, thread, pins, thimble, pattern	sewing tools
bottle, diaper, crib, formula, rattle	baby items
barn, silo, livestock, crops, tractor	farm words

> # FOCUS on MARRIAGE
> ## and FILL IN the BLANK.

1. Official documentation of a marriage is called a marriage **c**_____

2. The formal suit worn by the groom is a **t**_____

3. The exchange of wedding vows is part of the marriage

    c_____

4. The party following the marriage is the **r**_____

5. The young boy who carries the wedding bands is called the ring **b**_____

6. An old expression is "something old, something new, something borrowed and something **b**_____ "

7. The song traditionally played as the bride proceeds down the aisle is the "Wedding **M**_____ "

8. Following the wedding day, the newlyweds typically go on a **h**_____

9. When a woman accepts a man's proposal of marriage, the couple is said to be **e**_____

10. Unscramble these words (related to marriage):

    L E I V   _____

    T O Q U U E B   _____

    T A S O T   _____

    K C A E   _____

    G N R I   _____

ANSWERS TO:
FOCUS on <u>MARRIAGE</u>.

1. Official documentation of a marriage is called a marriage___certificate_____

2. The formal suit worn by the groom is a _tuxedo_____

3. The exchange of wedding vows is part of the marriage
   _____ceremony_____

4. The party following the marriage is the _reception_____

5. The young boy who carries the wedding bands is called the ring _bearer_____

6. An old expression is "something old, something new, something borrowed and something_blue_____"

7. The song traditionally played as the bride proceeds down the aisle is the "Wedding ____March_____"

8. Following the wedding day, the newlyweds typically go on a_honeymoon_____

9. When a woman accepts a man's proposal of marriage, the couple is said to be____engaged_____

10. Unscramble these words (related to marriage):

    L E I V _____veil_____

    T O Q U U E B _____bouquet_____

    T A S O T _____toast_____

    K C A E _____cake_____

    G N R I _____ring_____

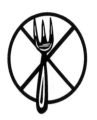

FILL IN the **BOX** with the **WORD THAT <u>DOESN'T BELONG</u>.** For example, "dog, cat, goldfish and hamster" are all pets; "fork" is NOT a pet—it doesn't belong in the group.

<u>ITEMS</u>	<u>DOESN'T BELONG</u>
dog, cat, fork, goldfish, hamster	fork
thread, scissors, needle, pattern, sifter	
gin, vodka, soda, bourbon, scotch	
mountain, highway, lake, river, valley	
car, van, jeep, canoe, SUV	
rain, sleet, wind, snow, hail	
in, above, under, now, behind	
bumpy, rough, happy, smooth, fuzzy	
always, hard, sometimes, now, never	
man, you, me, he, she	

ANSWERS TO:
FILL IN the BOX with the WORD THAT DOESN'T BELONG

ITEMS	DOESN'T BELONG
dog, cat, fork, goldfish, hamster	fork
thread, scissors, needle, pattern, sifter	sifter
gin, vodka, soda, bourbon, scotch	soda
mountain, highway, lake, river, valley	highway
car, van, jeep, canoe, SUV	canoe
rain, sleet, wind, snow, hail	wind
in, above, under, now, behind	now
bumpy, rough, happy, smooth, fuzzy	happy
always, hard, sometimes, now, never	hard
man, you, me, he, she	man

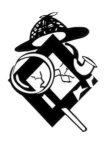

Use the clues to help you
NAME the **WORD**.

Clue	Answer
1. A sewing tool used to mend clothes	N _ _ _ _ _
2. Term for one piece of grass	B _ _ _ _ _
3. A feeling of hopelessness	D _ _ _ _ _ _
4. A prickly plant that grows in the desert	C _ _ _ _ _
5. The nut that squirrels gather	A _ _ _ _
6. What drops from an evergreen tree	P _ _ _ _ _ _
7. The sound associated with running brooks	B _ _ _ _ _ _
8. What covers the ground on the beach	S _ _ _
9. The flat land between two mountains	V _ _ _ _ _
10. What people like to gather on sandy beaches	S _ _ _ _ _

ANSWERS TO:
Use the clues to help you
NAME the **WORD**.

---

1. A sewing tool used to mend clothes	needle
2. Term for one piece of grass	blade
3. A feeling of hopelessness	despair
4. A prickly plant that grows in the desert	cactus
5. The nut that squirrels gather	acorn
6. What drops from an evergreen tree	pinecone
7. The sound associated with running brooks	babbling
8. What covers the ground on the beach	sand
9. The flat land between two mountains	valley
10. What people like to gather on sandy beaches	shells

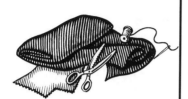

UNSCRAMBLE the **LETTERS** to make a word. HINT: All of the words are **FABRICS**. The first one is done for you.

N I L N E	L I N E N
T C T N O O	C _ _ _ _ _
T N S I A	S _ _ _ _
K S I L	S _ _ _
S P E D X N A	S _ _ _ _ _ _
A C Y L R C I	A _ _ _ _ _ _
L O W O	W _ _ _
R Y O C O U D R	C _ _ _ _ _ _ _
L M S U I N	M _ _ _ _ _
N L Y N O	N _ _ _ _

ANSWERS TO:
UNSCRAMBLE the
LETTERS to make a word.

N I L N E   <u>LINEN</u>

T C T N O O   <u>COTTON</u>

T N S I A   <u>SATIN</u>

K S I L   <u>SILK</u>

S P E D X N A   <u>SPANDEX</u>

A C Y L R C I   <u>ACRYLIC</u>

L O W O   <u>WOOL</u>

R Y O C O U D R   <u>CORDUROY</u>

L M S U I N   <u>MUSLIN</u>

N L Y N O   <u>NYLON</u>

PICTURE the DESCRIPTION, and then
FILL IN the BLANK.

1. I am the time of day when golden and red colors line the horizon. I am __s__

2. I am brilliant autumn leaves in New England, often termed fall __f__

3. I am formations of stars in the sky, like the "big dipper." I am called __c__

4. An imaginary line that divides the earth into Northern and Southern Hemispheres, I am the __e__

5. I am a machine that uses an air pump to suck up dust and dirt. I am a __v__

6. I am a portable electronic device used to perform basic and complex operations of arithmetic. I am a

   __c__

7. I am a very comfortable soft chair, with a foot rest, that can assume various positions. I am a __r__

8. I am a special type of twin beds, positioned one above the other. I am __b__

9. I am a type of canvas shoulder bag used by students to carry books. I am a __b__

10. I am a tool used to keep people dry from rain or cool from the sun's rays. I am an __u__

ANSWERS TO:
PICTURE the **DESCRIPTION**, and then
FILL IN the **BLANK**.

---

1. I am the time of day when golden and red colors line the horizon. I am <u> sunset   </u>

2. I am brilliant autumn leaves in New England, often termed fall <u> foliage   </u>

3. I am formations of stars in the sky, like the "big dipper." I am called <u> constellations   </u>

4. An imaginary line that divides the earth into Northern and Southern Hemispheres, I am the <u> equator   </u>

5. I am a machine that uses an air pump to suck up dust and dirt. I am a <u> vacuum cleaner   </u>

6. I am a portable electronic device used to perform basic and complex operations of arithmetic. I am a

   <u> calculator   </u>

7. I am a very comfortable soft chair, with a foot rest, that can assume various positions. I am a <u> recliner   </u>

8. I am a special type of twin beds, positioned one above the other. I am <u>bunk beds   </u>

9. I am a type of canvas shoulder bag used by students to carry books. I am a <u> back pack   </u>

10. I am a tool used to keep people dry from rain or cool from the sun's rays. I am an <u> umbrella   </u>

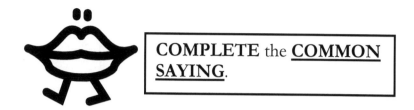

COMPLETE the COMMON SAYING.

1. When a student copies the work of another, they may be called a " _____ "

2. Someone who works very hard might be described as an "eager _____ "

3. A no-win situation is sometimes termed a catch "____ "

4. People who need a nap might say that they want to "catch forty _____ "

5. An item that is cheap and common can be described as "a dime a _____ "

6. When you look great, you might be told you "look like a million _____ "

7. When a student skips school when they're supposed to go, they're accused of "playing _____ "

8. If very happy about something, you might be described a being "on cloud _____ "

9. You're likely to want to help someone who has helped you because "one good turn deserves _____ "

10. If you want to add your opinion to a discussion you might ask permission to "put in your two _____ "

ANSWERS TO: COMPLETE the COMMON SAYING.

1. When a student copies the work of another, they may be called a " copy cat "

2. Someone who works very hard might be described as an "eager beaver "

3. A no-win situation is sometimes termed a "catch 22 "

4. People who need a nap might say that they want to "catch forty winks "

5. An item that is cheap and common can be described as "a dime a dozen "

6. When you look great, you might be told you "look like a million dollars "

7. When a student skips school when they're supposed to go, they're accused of "playing hooky "

8. If very happy about something, you might be described a being "on cloud nine "

9. You're likely to want to help someone who has helped you because "one good turn deserves another "

10. If you want to add your opinion to a discussion you might ask permission to "put in your two cents "

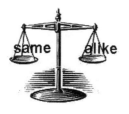

FILL IN the box with a **SYNONYM,** a word that **MEANS THE SAME**. For example, "rich" and "wealthy" are synonyms.

RICH	WEALTHY
HORS D'OEURVRE	
PETITE	
ROBBER	
BRAVE	
SLIM	
COUCH	
SOUR	
ELDERLY	
RUG	
HOMELY	

ANSWERS TO:
FILL IN the box with a
SYNONYM.

RICH	WEALTHY
HORS D'OEURVRE	APPETIZER
PETITE	SHORT
ROBBER	THIEF
BRAVE	COURAGEOUS
SLIM	THIN
COUCH	SOFA
SOUR	TART
ELDERLY	OLD
RUG	CARPET
HOMELY	UGLY

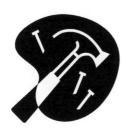

NAME the **ACTION** or **USE** of the **OBJECT**. For example, we tap a hammer.

HAMMER	TAP
KNIFE	
MARACAS	
TWEEZERS	
SPATULA	
STATIONERY	
CHAIR	
TWINE	
BATON	
BED	
SEEDS	

ANSWERS TO:
NAME the **ACTION** or
USE of the **OBJECT**.

HAMMER	TAP
KNIFE	CUT
MARACAS	SHAKE
TWEEZERS	PLUCK
SPATULA	WIPE
STATIONERY	WRITE ON
CHAIR	SIT ON
TWINE	TIE, WRAP
BATON	TWIRL
BED	SLEEP ON
SEEDS	PLANT

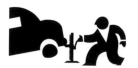

NAME the **ACTIVITY**, given the **TOOLS**. The first one is done for you.

jack, lug wrench, spare	change a flat tire
passport, airline tickets, foreign currency, itinerary	
bedding, clothes, money, meal plan, books, computer	
alley, heavy ball, ten pins, scorecard, shoes	
snowsuit, boots, hat, mittens, coal, broom, carrot, sticks, scarf	
toothpaste, toothbrush, pajamas or nightgown, soap, water, towel	
vacuum, Windex, furniture polish, mop, dust cloths, paper towels	
ladder, chain saw, cherry picker, wood chipper	
nine hoops in the ground, mallets, wooden balls	
9-volt battery, step stool	

<u>ANSWERS TO:</u>
NAME the **<u>ACTIVITY</u>,**
given the **TOOLS.**

jack, lug wrench, spare	change a flat tire
passport, airline tickets, foreign currency, itinerary	travel abroad
bedding, clothes, money, meal plan, books, computer	start in college
alley, heavy ball, ten pins, scorecard, shoes	go bowling
snowsuit, boots, hat, mittens, coal, broom, carrot, sticks, scarf	make a snowman
toothpaste, toothbrush, pajamas or nightgown, soap, water, towel	get ready for bed
vacuum, Windex, furniture polish, mop, dust cloths, paper towels	clean house
ladder, chain saw, cherry picker, wood chipper	chop down tree
nine hoops in the ground, mallets, wooden balls	play croquet
9-volt battery, step stool	replace smoke detector battery

NAME the **OCCUPATION**, given the "tools of the trade." The first one is done for you.

ladder, hydrant, ax, extinguisher, hose	firefighter
tall white chair, rescue buoy or ring, tow line, first aid kit	
stamps, money drawer, packing tape, scale	
air pump, oil can, fuel pump, windshield cleaner	
polish, rags, sponges, wax, brushes	
hangers, coat rack, tip dish, tickets	
shaker, strainer, glasses, liquor, blender, ice chipper	
tape measure, pins, marking chalk, mirror, sewing machine	
studio, teleprompter, make-up artist, dressing room, maps, microphone	
Petrie dishes, test tubes centrifuge, microscope	

ANSWERS TO:
NAME the **OCCUPATION**,
given the "tools of the trade."

ladder, hydrant, ax, extinguisher, hose	firefighter
tall white chair, rescue buoy or ring, tow line, first aid kit	lifeguard
stamps, money drawer, packing tape, scale	postal clerk
air pump, oil can, fuel pump, windshield cleaner	gas station attendant
polish, rags, sponges, wax, brushes	housekeeper
hangers, coat rack, tip dish, tickets	coat checker
shaker, strainer, glasses, liquor, blender, ice chipper	bartender
tape measure, pins, marking chalk, mirror, sewing machine	seamstress or tailor
studio, teleprompter, make-up artist, dressing room, maps, microphone	meteorologist
Petrie dishes, test tubes centrifuge, microscope	chemist

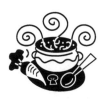

NAME the **FOOD** or **BEVERAGE,** given the ingredients and tools. The first one is done for you.

broth, egg noodles, vegetables, salt, pepper, seasonings	vegetable soup
cheese, onions, milk, salt & pepper, eggs, chopped ham or bacon, frying pan	
onion, eggs, shredded potatoes, flour, salt & pepper, oil	
OJ & champagne	
bread, eggs, cinnamon, milk, syrup, butter	
wide pasta, ricotta, mozzarella, eggs, ground beef, tomatoes, tomato paste, Italian seasoning	
bread crumbs or cubes, onions, water, poultry seasoning, butter	
French bread, tomatoes, fresh basil, oregano & garlic, mozzarella, olive oil	
lettuce, cucumber, tomatoes, olives, dressing	

ANSWERS TO: NAME the FOOD or BEVERAGE.	

broth, egg noodles, vegetables, salt, pepper, seasonings	vegetable soup
cheese, onions, milk, salt & pepper, eggs, chopped ham or bacon, frying pan	omelette
onion, eggs, shredded potatoes, flour, salt & pepper, oil	potato latkes
OJ & champagne	mimosa
bread, eggs, cinnamon, milk, syrup, butter	French toast
wide pasta, ricotta, mozzarella, eggs, ground beef, tomatoes, tomato paste, Italian seasoning	lasagna
bread crumbs or cubes, onions, water, poultry seasoning, butter	stuffing
French bread, tomatoes, fresh basil, oregano & garlic, mozzarella, olive oil	bruschetta
lettuce, cucumber, tomatoes, olives, dressing	salad

> ### NAME the FAMOUS LOCATION.

1. The capital of Italy and home of the Vatican is_____

2. A famous hiking trail in Eastern US is the _____

3. The volcanic eruption that destroyed Pompeii occurred on Mount _____

4. Many tourists are determined to kiss the Blarney Stone in _____

5. One of the oldest cities in the world and a holy city to three religions is _____

6. Part of the coast of France, a resort area for the rich and famous, is the French _____

7. The district of Los Angeles considered the center of movie studios and movie stars is _____

8. The oldest city in the United States is _____

9. The Mayflower Pilgrims first landed at _____

10. Davy Crockett took part in the Texas Revolution and was killed at the Battle of the_____

ANSWERS TO: NAME the FAMOUS LOCATION.

1. The capital of Italy and home of the Vatican is_Rome_

2. A famous hiking trail in Eastern US is the Appalachian

3. The volcanic eruption that destroyed Pompeii occurred on Mount Vesuvius

4. Many tourists are determined to kiss the Blarney Stone in Ireland

5. One of the oldest cities in the world and a holy city to three religions is Jerusalem

6. Part of the coast of France, a resort area for the rich and famous, is the French Riviera

7. The district of Los Angeles considered the center of movie studios and movie stars is Hollywood

8. The oldest city in the United States is St. Augustine

9. The Mayflower Pilgrims first landed at Plymouth Rock

10. Davy Crockett took part in the Texas Revolution and was killed at the Battle of the Alamo

???

FILL IN the **BLANK** to **IDENTIFY** a **PERSON**. Note: There may be more than one correct answer.

1. Rich folks often employ a driver, also called their personal _____

2. A man's servant is called his _____

3. A domestic assistant from a foreign country is called an _____

4. Robin Hood stole from the rich to support the _____

5. A person with a prominent profile with much public attention is a _____

6. An actor/actress who wins the academy award is often called a movie _____

7. An American pioneer, born on a mountaintop in Tennessee, was _____

8. Thomas Jefferson sent two men to explore the new west, namely, Lewis and _____

9. The woman credited with making the first American flag is _____

10. A person who claims to be able to predict another person's life is a _____

> ## ANSWERS TO:
> ## FILL IN the BLANK to
> ## IDENTIFY a PERSON.

1. Rich folks often employ a driver, also called their personal ___chauffeur___

2. A man's servant is called his ___valet___

3. A domestic assistant from a foreign country is called an ___au pair___

4. Robin Hood stole from the rich to support the _poor_

5. A person with a prominent profile with much public attention is a ___celebrity___

6. An actor/actress who wins the academy award is often called a movie ___star___

7. An American pioneer, born on a mountaintop in Tennessee, was ___Davy Crockett___

8. Thomas Jefferson sent two men to explore the new west, namely, Lewis and ___Clark___

9. The woman credited with making the first American flag is ___Betsy Ross___

10. A person who claims to be able to predict another person's life is a ___fortune teller or soothsayer___

???

FILL IN the **BLANK** to **IDENTIFY** an **OBJECT**. Note: There may be more than one correct answer.

1. Another name for a trash can is a _____

2. The tool used for sweeping is a _____

3. When autumn leaves fall, you may need to take out your _____

4. Children love to build towers with _____

5. Ice hockey players hit a round disc called a_____

6. In a fairy tale, Jack climbed a tall plant called a _____

7. In another tale, Jack jumped over the _____

8. In yet another tale, Jack and Jill climbed up a _____

9. On a windy day, you may opt to fly a _____

10. We can improve our vision by wearing _____

> ## ANSWERS TO:
> ## FILL IN the BLANK to
> ## IDENTIFY an OBJECT.

1. Another name for a trash can is a <u>garbage can</u>

2. The tool used for sweeping is a <u>broom</u>

3. When autumn leaves fall, you may need to take out your <u>rake</u>

4. Children love to build towers with <u>blocks</u>

5. Ice hockey players hit a round disc called a <u>puck</u>

6. In a fairy tale, Jack climbed a tall plant called a <u>bean stalk</u>

7. In another tale, Jack jumped over the <u>candlestick</u>

8. In yet another tale, Jack and Jill climbed up a <u>hill</u>

9. On a windy day, you may opt to fly a <u>kite</u>

10. We can improve our vision by wearing <u>glasses</u>

??? | **FILL IN** the **BLANK** to **IDENTIFY** a **PLACE**. Note: There may be more than one correct answer.

1. Teachers typically eat lunch in the teacher's _____

2. City dwellers often enjoy taking a walk in the _____

3. In olden days, prisoners were hung on a _____

4. People stroll along city streets on a cement path called a _____

5. U.S. tourists who need information about local accommodations and happenings might stop at the

   _____

6. Working parents might take their toddlers to a

   _____

7. People often grow flowers and crops in a _____

8. Yachts are often kept at a slip in a _____

9. Children in grade school usually enjoy their recess on a

   _____

10. When you go the emergency room, you are likely to have to spend some time in the _____

> ## ANSWERS TO:
> ## FILL IN the BLANK to
> ## IDENTIFY a PLACE.

1. Teachers typically eat lunch in the teacher's __lounge__

2. City dwellers often enjoy taking a walk in the __park__

3. In olden days, prisoners were hung on a __gallows__

4. People stroll along city streets on a cement path called a _____ sidewalk _____

5. U.S. tourists who need information about local accommodations and happenings might stop at the _____ visitor's center _____

6. Working parents might take their toddlers to a _____ day care center _____

7. People often grow flowers and crops in a __garden__

8. Yachts are often kept at a slip in a __marina or harbor__

9. Children in grade school usually enjoy their recess on a _____ playground _____

10. When you go the emergency room, you are likely to have to spend some time in the _____ waiting room _____

???

> Think about **TIME OR EVENTS** and **FILL IN** the **BLANK**. Note: There may be more than one correct answer.

1. The final competition in professional football in the US takes place on _____

2. Restaurants offer discounts on dinner during their early bird _____

3. Celebrations ending on the day before Ash Wednesday are called _____

4. The final competition of the professional baseball season in the U.S. is called the _____

5. Young people in the U.S. who turn 16 years of age become eligible to obtain a _____

6. At the age of three, toddlers in the U.S. typically begin _____

7. When people in the U.S. reach the age of 65, they often think of entering a stage of life called _____

8. Children typically being public education in the U.S. at the age of five, when they enter _____

9. Young people entering a trade might serve a period of time working under a licensed professional ... that time period is an _____

> ## ANSWERS TO:
> Think about **TIME OR EVENTS** and **FILL IN** the **BLANK**.

1. The final competition in professional football in the US takes place on ___Super Bowl Sunday___

2. Restaurants offer discounts on dinner during their early bird ___specials___

3. Celebrations ending on the day before Ash Wednesday are called ___Mardi Gras___

4. The final competition of the professional baseball season in the U.S. is called the ___World Series___

5. Young people in the U.S. who turn 16 years of age become eligible to obtain a ___driver's license___

6. At the age of three, toddlers in the U.S. typically begin ___preschool___

7. When people in the U.S. reach the age of 65, they often think of entering a stage of life called ___retirement___

8. Children typically being public education in the U.S. at the age of five, when they enter ___kindergarten___

9. Young people entering a trade might serve a period of time working under a licensed professional ... that time period is an ___apprenticeship___

> **THINK ABOUT REASONS WE DO THINGS** and **FILL IN** the **BLANK.** Note: There may be more than one correct answer.

1. People with sinus problems may use a nasal spray with a salty or _____ solution.

2. To get the job done more quickly, you may opt to use a _____ when painting walls.

3. Countries impose special checks on visitors crossing their borders to ensure against _____ entry.

4. To be certain we put proper ingredients into a dish, we use a cookbook and follow a _____

5. If we wear shoes that are too small, our feet may develop sores called _____

6. When we notice white spots on colored clothing, we may suspect an inadvertent splash of _____

7. When you can no longer button your trousers, you may suspect that you have gained a bit of _____

8. If your car stops unexpectedly, you may realize that you have run out of _____

9. Police sometimes use fingerprints to identify the suspect in a _____

10. When people move to a new home, they typically advise the post office of a _____ address

ANSWERS TO:
THINK ABOUT REASONS
WE DO THINGS and FILL IN
the BLANK.

1. People with sinus problems may use a nasal spray with a salty or ___saline___ solution.

2. To get the job done more quickly, you may opt to use a ___roller___ when painting walls.

3. Countries impose special checks on visitors crossing their borders to ensure against ___illegal___ entry.

4. To be certain we put proper ingredients into a dish, we use a cookbook and follow a ___recipe___

5. If we wear shoes that are too small, our feet may develop sores called ___blisters___

6. When we notice white spots on colored clothing, we may suspect an inadvertent splash of ___bleach___

7. When you can no longer button your trousers, you may suspect that you have gained a bit of ___weight___

8. If your car stops unexpectedly, you may realize that you have run out of ___gas or fuel___

9. Police sometimes use fingerprints to identify the suspect in a ___crime___

10. When people move to a new home, they typically advise the post office of a ___forwarding___ address.

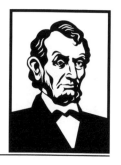

CIRCLE the **NAMES OF PRESIDENTS** that appear on the 3 lists below. You should find 15 presidents all together. Good luck!

List 1	List 2	List 3
James	Clinton	Madison
Ford	Churchill	Dole
Rockefeller	Roosevelt	Adams
Eisenhower	Reagan	Marshall
Washington	Stevenson	Grant
Lincoln	Kennedy	Polk
Cheney	Bush	Smith
Truman	Quayle	Wheeler
Harrison	Anderson	Patterson
Calhoun	Wilson	Obama

ANSWERS TO:
CIRCLE the NAMES
OF 15 PRESIDENTS.

List 1	List 2	List 3
	Clinton	Madison
Ford		
	Roosevelt	Adams
Eisenhower	Reagan	
Washington		Grant
Lincoln	Kennedy	Polk
	Bush	
Harrison		
		Obama

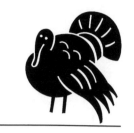

NAME 10 FOODS
associated with
THANKSGIVING
DINNER. HINT: Think of
meat, vegetables, and

1. _____

2. _____

3. _____

4. _____

5. _____

6. _____

7. _____

8. _____

9. _____

10. _____

<u>ANSWERS TO:</u>
NAME 10 FOODS
associated with
<u>THANKSGIVING</u>
<u>DINNER.</u>

1. turkey

2. gravy

3. stuffing

4. cranberry sauce

5. creamed onions

6. sweet potatoes

7. mashed potatoes

8. green beans

9. dinner rolls

10. pumpkin pie

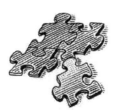

> **READ** the **ITEMS**; then **NAME** the <u>**CATEGORY**</u>. For example, "dog, cat, bird, goldfish and hamster" go together because they belong to the category of "pets."

<u>ITEMS</u>	<u>CATEGORY</u>
dog, cat, bird, goldfish, hamster	pets
conductor, engineer, tracks, tickets, schedule	
tissue, vaporizer, rest, Vitamin C, aspirin	
balloons, streamers, goody bags, games, cake	
blanket, sunscreen, umbrella, towels, bathing suit	
toilet, bathtub, sink, medicine chest, towels	
mask, tank, fins, snorkel, wet suit	
shrimp cocktail, cheese & crackers, chips and dips, nuts	
wrapping paper, scissors, tape, ribbon	

ANSWERS TO:
NAME the **CATEGORY**.

ITEMS	CATEGORY
dog, cat, bird, goldfish, hamster	pets
conductor, engineer, tracks, tickets, schedule	train items
tissue, vaporizer, rest, Vitamin C, aspirin	help for a cold
balloons, streamers, goody bags, games, cake	birthday party
blanket, sunscreen, umbrella, towels, bathing suit	things for the beach
toilet, bathtub, sink, medicine chest, towels	bathroom items
mask, tank, fins, snorkel, wet suit	scuba gear
shrimp cocktail, cheese & crackers, chips and dips, nuts	appetizers
wrapping paper, scissors, tape, ribbon	things to wrap a gift

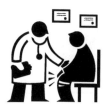

FOCUS on the **DOCTOR** and **FILL IN** the **BLANK**.

1. The date/time of a visit is called an **a** _____

2. After checking in, patients are usually told to have a seat in the **w** _____ **r** _____

3. The nurse takes your temperature with a

   t _____

4. The nurse checks your heart function by taking your

   b _____ **p** _____

5. The nurse usually asks for a list of the pills you are taking, called your " **m** _____ "

6. The doctor reviews your medical history and records new information in your medical **c** _____

7. When you need new medication, the doctor gives you a

   p _____

8. The doctor listens to your breathing with a **s** _____

9. Unscramble these words (related to the doctor):

   N A B D A G E   _____

   D E E E N L   _____

   C S A L E   _____

   Y P S H A I C L   _____

   F X E R O L S E   _____

ANSWERS TO:
FOCUS on the **DOCTOR**
and **FILL IN** the **BLANK**.

---

1. The date/time of a visit is called an _appointment_

2. After checking in, patients are usually told to have a seat in the _waiting_ _room_

3. The nurse takes your temperature with a
thermometer

4. The nurse checks your heart function by taking your
blood _pressure_

5. The nurse usually asks for a list of the pills you are taking, called your "_medications_"

6. The doctor reviews your medical history and records new information in your medical _chart_

7. When you need new medication, the doctor gives you a
prescription

8. The doctor listens to your breathing with a _stethoscope_

9. Unscramble these words (related to the doctor):

    N A B D A G E   _bandage_

    D E E E N L   _needle_

    C S A L E   _scale_

    Y P S H A I C L   _physical_

    F X E R O L S E   _flexors_

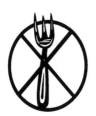

FILL IN the BOX with the WORD THAT DOESN'T BELONG. For example, "dog, cat, goldfish and hamster" are all pets; "fork" is NOT a pet—it doesn't belong in the group.

ITEMS	DOESN'T BELONG
dog, cat, fork, goldfish, hamster	fork
Nile, Mississippi, Ganges, Rockies, Amazon	
concert, orchestra, theatre, choir, chorus	
dictator, secretary, king, president, queen	
raccoon, ape, orangutan, chimp, gorilla	
nail, screw, toothpick, bolt, nut	
stomach, heart, arteries, veins, capillaries	
addition, eviction, subtraction, multiplication, division	
German, Spanish, Scotch, English, French	
office, home, abode, domicile, house	

> ## ANSWERS TO:
> ## FILL IN the BOX with the WORD
> ## THAT DOESN'T BELONG.

ITEMS	DOESN'T BELONG
dog, cat, fork, goldfish, hamster	fork
Nile, Mississippi, Ganges, Rockies, Amazon	Rockies
concert, orchestra, theatre, choir, chorus	theatre
dictator, secretary, king, president, queen	secretary
raccoon, ape, orangutan, chimp, gorilla	raccoon
nail, screw, toothpick, bolt, nut	toothpick
stomach, heart, arteries, veins, capillaries	stomach
addition, eviction, subtraction, multiplication, division	eviction
German, Spanish, Scotch, English, French	Scotch
office, home, abode, domicile, house	office

Use the clues to help you
NAME the **WORD**.

1. The bright circle of light above an angel's head	H _ _ _ _
2. The sound made by an ambulance or police car	S _ _ _ _
3. A tightly rolled bundle of tobacco ignited so its smoke is drawn into the mouth	C _ _ _ _
4. The eventful dance for juniors and seniors in high school	P _ _ _
5. A purple variety of quartz used in jewelry	A _ _ _ _ _ _
6. The headwear worn at graduation	C _ _
7. The certificate issued at high school graduation	D _ _ _ _ _ _
8. The award given to the best movie	O _ _ _ _
9. An entrance through a fence	G _ _ _
10. Abbreviation for an underwater navy vessel	S _ _

> ## ANSWERS TO:
> Use the clues to help you
> ## NAME the WORD.

1. The bright circle of light above an angel's head	halo
2. The sound made by an ambulance or police car	siren
3. A tightly rolled bundle of tobacco ignited so its smoke is drawn into the mouth	cigar
4. The eventful dance for juniors and seniors in high school	prom
5. A purple variety of quartz used in jewelry	amethyst
6. The headwear worn at graduation	cap
7. The certificate issued at high school graduation	diploma
8. The award given to the best movie	Oscar
9. An entrance through a fence	gate
10. Abbreviation for an underwater navy vessel	sub

> **UNSCRAMBLE** the **LETTERS** to make a word. HINT: All of the words are **THINGS THAT FLY**. The first one is done for you.

DRIB   B I R D

TIEK   K _ _ _

NLPAE   P _ _ _ _

KUCD   D _ _ _

OOGSE   G _ _ _ _

PLBMI   B _ _ _ _

GLFA   F _ _ _

PWAS   W _ _ _

GLEEA   E _ _ _ _

SOREPY   O _ _ _ _ _

ANSWERS TO:
UNSCRAMBLE the
LETTERS to make a word.

D R I B   **BIRD**

T I E K   **KITE**

N L P A E   **PLANE**

K U C D   **DUCK**

O O G S E   **GOOSE**

P L B M I   **BLIMP**

G L F A   **FLAG**

P W A S   **WASP**

G L E E A   **EAGLE**

S O R E P Y   **OSPREY**

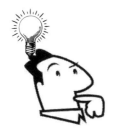

PICTURE the DESCRIPTION;
then FILL IN the BLANK.

1. I am lenses placed directly on the eyes to correct vision. I am _____

2. I am a specialty store that sells a variety of meat and cheese sandwiches. I am a _____

3. I am a type of earring worn through a hole in the earlobe. I am a _____

4. I am a small plate that supports a cup. I am a_____

5. I am a flowering weed with yellow blossoms that open during the day and close at night. I am a _____

6. I am an annual publication with information about weather, tides and planting times. I am a Farmer's

_____

7. I am a dummy used to display fashions in department stores and store windows. I am a _____

8. I am a tropical marine animal whose hard skeleton is important in coastal reefs. I am _____

9. I am a colorful wax writing implement used by children to color. I am a_____

10. I am a round operating mechanism turned to secure and open a door. I am a _____

ANSWERS TO:
PICTURE the DESCRIPTION

1. I am lenses placed directly on the eyes to correct vision.
   I am _____contacts_____

2. I am a specialty store that sells a variety of meat and
   cheese sandwiches. I am a _____delicatessen_____

3. I am a type of earring worn through a hole in the
   earlobe. I am a _____pierced earring_____

4. I am a small plate that supports a cup. I am a_saucer_

5. I am a flowering weed with yellow blossoms that open
   during the day and close at night. I am a _dandelion___

6. I am an annual publication with information about
   weather, tides and planting times. I am a Farmer's

   _____Almanac_____

7. I am a dummy used to display fashions in department
   stores and store windows. I am a _mannequin_____

8. I am a tropical marine animal whose hard skeleton is
   important in coastal reefs. I am _____coral_____

9. I am a colorful wax writing implement used by children
   to color. I am a_____crayon_____

10. I am a round operating mechanism turned to secure
    and open a door. I am a _____lock_____

COMPLETE the COMMON SAYING.

1. When a person gets into trouble, they might say, "My goose is _____"

2. A very small amount of money might be described as "chicken _____"

3. A person who is confused in a crowd might feel like they're "lost in the _____"

4. Someone who is mentally deficient might be described as "not playing with a full _____"

5. A person who feels very healthy might say, "I'm on top of the _____"

7. People wearing their finest clothing are "dressed to _____"

6. A very strong person is "as strong as an _____"

8. Very thick fog might be described as being "as thick as _____"

9. If you behaved in a very crazy way, friends might way you "went off your _____"

10. Someone who loves candy, desserts and sweets has a real "sweet _____"

> ## ANSWERS TO:
> ## COMPLETE the COMMON
> ## SAYING.

1. When a person gets into trouble, they might say, "My goose is ___cooked___ "

2. A very small amount of money might be described as "chicken ___feed___ "

3. A person who is confused in a crowd might feel like they're "lost in the ___shuffle___ "

4. Someone who is mentally deficient might be described as "not playing with a full ___deck___ "

5. A person who feels very healthy might say, "I'm on top of the ___world___ "

7. People wearing their finest clothing are "dressed to ___kill___ "

6. A very strong person is "as strong as an ___ox___ "

8. Very thick fog might be described as being "as thick as ___pea soup___ "

9. If you behaved in a very crazy way, friends might way you "went off your ___rocker___ "

10. Someone who loves candy, desserts and sweets has a real "sweet ___tooth___ "

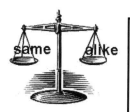

FILL IN the box with a **SYNONYM,** a word that **MEANS THE SAME**. For example, "rich" and "wealthy" are synonyms.

RICH	**WEALTHY**
ROBBER	
BABY	
"JOCK"	
SHIP	
BEVERAGE	
GIFT	
GLAD	
HOMELY	
HUGE	
LOFTY	

ANSWERS TO:
FILL IN the box with a
SYNONYM.

RICH	WEALTHY
CLIFF	PRECIPICE
BABY	INFANT
"JOCK"	ATHLETE
SHIP	VESSEL
BEVERAGE	DRINK
GIFT	PRESENT
GLAD	HAPPY
UGLY	UNATTRACTIVE
HUGE	GIGANTIC
LOFTY	HIGH

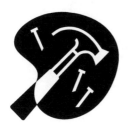

NAME the **ACTION** or **USE** of the **OBJECT**. For example, we tap a hammer.

HAMMER	TAP
SPOON	
KEY	
AX	
HOSE	
NEEDLE	
YARN	
ENVELOPE	
WREATH	
SCALE	
TISSUE	

ANSWERS TO:
NAME the **ACTION** or
USE of the **OBJECT**.

HAMMER	TAP
SPOON	STIR OR MIX
KEY	LOCK OR UNLOCK
AX	CHOP
HOSE	SPRAY OR WATER
NEEDLE	SEW OR MEND
YARN	KNIT
ENVELOPE	MAIL OR SEND
WREATH	HANG
SCALE	WEIGH
TISSUE	BLOW OR WIPE

NAME the **ACTIVITY**, given the **TOOLS**. The first one is done for you.	
jack, lug wrench, spare	change a flat tire
veil, gown, bouquet, limo	
bat, mitt, bases, ball	
jars/lids, pot of boiling water, pectin, fruit, masher, sugar	
clean outfit, backpack, lunchbox, books, homework	
clubs, balls, bag, cart, shoes	
tractor, flatbed trailer, apple orchard, camera	
helmet, shoulder and knee pads, ball, goal and yard lines	
heavy coat, boots, gloves, shovel	
corsage, fancy dress, date, dancing shoes, limo	
table with 4 chairs, deck of 48 cards, scorecard, pencil	

<table>
<tr><td colspan="2"><u>ANSWERS TO:</u>
NAME the ACTIVITY,
given the TOOLS.</td></tr>
</table>

jack, lug wrench, spare	change a flat tire
veil, gown, bouquet, limo	get married
bat, mitt, bases, ball	play baseball
jars/lids, pot of boiling water, pectin, fruit, masher, sugar	can jam or jelly
clean outfit, backpack, lunchbox, books, homework	go to school
clubs, balls, bag, cart, shoes	play golf
tractor, flatbed trailer, apple orchard, camera	go on a hayride
helmet, shoulder and knee pads, ball, goal and yard lines	play football
heavy coat, boots, gloves, shovel	shovel snow
corsage, fancy dress, date, dancing shoes, limo	go to prom
table with 4 chairs, deck of 48 cards, scorecard, pencil	play pinochle

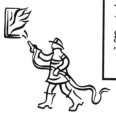

NAME the **OCCUPATION**, given the "tools of the trade." The first one is done for you.

ladder, hydrant, ax, extinguisher, hose	firefighter
flippers, air tank, mask, wet suit, regulator	
leaf blower, weed whacker, mower, rake	
hard-hat, jack-hammer, pay loader, truck	
livery license, cell phone, change, Lincoln Town Car	
revolver, cruiser, handcuffs, billy club, badge	
comb, brush, shampoo, towel, scissors, dryer	
car lift, pneumatic tools, grease/oil, coveralls	
vault, money drawer, forms, computers	
foliage, trimmer, tape, foam, flora, vase, wire	

<u>ANSWERS TO</u>:
NAME the **<u>OCCUPATION</u>,**
given the "tools of the trade."

ladder, hydrant, ax, extinguisher, hose	firefighter
flippers, air tank, mask, wet suit, regulator	scuba diver
leaf blower, weed whacker, mower, rake	landscaper
hard-hat, jack-hammer, pay loader, truck	construction worker
livery license, cell phone, change, Lincoln Town Car	chauffeur
revolver, cruiser, handcuffs, billy club, badge	police officer
comb, brush, shampoo, towel, scissors, dryer	hairdresser barber
car lift, pneumatic tools, grease/oil, coveralls	auto mechanic
vault, money drawer, forms, computers	banker
foliage, trimmer, tape, foam, flora, vase, wire	florist

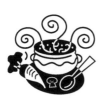

NAME the **FOOD** or **BEVERAGE,** given the ingredients and tools. The first one is done for you.

broth, egg noodles, vegetables, salt, pepper, seasonings	vegetable soup
cream cheese, sour cream, sugar, eggs, milk, vanilla, crust	
beef, carrots, potatoes, onion, oil, water, seasonings, celery	
onions, white wine, oil, beef chuck, sour cream, flour, beef broth, noodles, mushrooms	
shredded cabbage, grated carrots, vinegar, sugar, mayo, onion, S&P	
dark rye bread, corned beef, Swiss cheese, sauerkraut, dressing	
elbow pasta, cheese, flour, milk, butter, pepper	
crepes, cottage cheese, egg yolks, sugar, lemon juice, oil	
long/thin pasta, tomato sauce, meatballs, parmesan cheese	

```
┌─────────────────────────────┐
│      ANSWERS TO:            │
│  NAME the FOOD or           │
│  BEVERAGE, given the        │
│  ingredients and tools      │
└─────────────────────────────┘
```

broth, egg noodles, vegetables, salt, pepper, seasonings	vegetable soup
cream cheese, sour cream, sugar, eggs, milk, vanilla, crust	cheesecake
beef, carrots, potatoes, onion, oil, water, seasonings, celery	stew
onions, white wine, oil, beef chuck, sour cream, flour, beef broth, noodles, mushrooms	beef stroganoff
shredded cabbage, grated carrots, vinegar, sugar, mayo, onion, S&P	coleslaw
dark rye bread, corned beef, Swiss cheese, sauerkraut, dressing	reuben
elbow pasta, cheese, flour, milk, butter, pepper	mac & cheese
crepes, cottage cheese, egg yolks, sugar, lemon juice, oil	blintzes
long/thin pasta, tomato sauce, meatballs, parmesan cheese	spaghetti

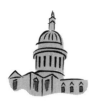

NAME the FAMOUS LOCATION.

1. The longest river in the world is the _____

2. The wetlands covering a large part of Southern Florida are the _____

3. The barrier built in Germany to prevent East Germans from defecting after WWII was the_____

4. The highest mountain in Africa is _____

5. The large neighborhood in the northern part of Manhattan, known as a major African-American center, is _____

6. The western-most city in Mexico, nicknamed the "Gateway to Mexico," is _____

7. The northern-most point on the earth is the _____

8. The longest river in South America is the _____

9. Columbus first sailed westward to gain access to the spice trade in the _____

10. A historic castle on the River Thames in London, which was also used as a prison, is the _____

ANSWERS TO: NAME the FAMOUS LOCATION.

1. The longest river in the world is the _____ Nile _____

2. The wetlands covering a large part of Southern Florida are the ___ Everglades _____

3. The barrier built in Germany to prevent East Germans from defecting after WWII was the Berlin Wall _____

4. The highest mountain in Africa is ___ Kilimanjaro _____

5. The large neighborhood in the northern part of Manhattan, known as a major African-American center, is _____ Harlem _____

6. The western-most city in Mexico, nicknamed the "Gateway to Mexico," is ___ Tijuana _____

7. The northern-most point on earth is the ___ North Pole

8. The longest river in South America is the ___ Amazon ___

9. Columbus first sailed westward to gain access to the spice trade in the _____ West Indies _____

10. A historic castle on the River Thames in London, which was also used as a prison, is the Tower of London _____

???

> **FILL IN** the **BLANK** to
> **IDENTIFY** a **PERSON**.
> Note: There may be more
> than one correct answer.

1. The original people who inhabit a land are the_____

2. People who move from their homeland and settle in a new country are _____

3. Beings reputed to come from outer space are _____

4. The person who manages a circus performance is the

   _____

5. The highest ranking officer in the army is a _____

6. The highest ranking officer in the navy is an _____

7. The player who calls the plays in a football game is the

   _____

8. A person who monitors prisoners after their release is a

   _____

9. A corrections officer in charge of a prison is a _____

10. A minister in a specialized setting, such as a prison, hospital or military unit is called a _____

ANSWERS TO:
FILL IN the **BLANK** to
IDENTIFY a **PERSON**.

---

1. The original people who inhabit a land are __natives__

2. People who move from their homeland and settle in a new country are ___emigrants or immigrants___

3. Beings reputed to come from outer space are _aliens_

4. The person who manages a circus performance is the ____ringmaster____

5. The highest ranking officer in the army is a _general_

6. The highest ranking officer in the navy is an _admiral_

7. The player who calls the plays in a football game is the ____quarterback____

8. A person who monitors prisoners after their release is a ____parole or probation officer____

9. A corrections officer in charge of a prison is a _warden_

10. A minister in a specialized setting, such as a prison, hospital or military unit is called a ____chaplain____

??? FILL IN the BLANK to IDENTIFY an OBJECT.
Note: There may be more than one correct answer.

1. The vertical brick structure that vents smoke from a fireplace is a _____

2. An insect that changes into a butterfly is a _____

3. A large outdoor fire used as part of a celebration is a

   _____

4. A countertop electrical slow cooker is a _____

5. Seamstresses often store their pins in a pin _____

6. The highest court in the US is the_____

7. Any substance that is involved in causing cancer is a

   _____

8. The heavy metal previously used in household paint and construction, which has been found to have harmful effects on humans, is _____

9. Bushes that adorn the front of homes are called

   _____

10. A face covering worn for disguise or performance is
    a _____

> ## ANSWERS TO:
> ### FILL IN the BLANK to IDENTIFY an OBJECT.

1. The vertical brick structure that vents smoke from a fireplace is a _____chimney_____

2. An insect that changes into a butterfly is a _caterpillar_

3. A large outdoor fire used as part of a celebration is a _____bonfire_____

4. A countertop electrical slow cooker is a ___crock pot___

5. Seamstresses often store their pins in a pin _cushion_

6. The highest court in the US is the__Supreme Court__

7. Any substance that is involved in causing cancer is a _____carcinogen_____

8. The heavy metal previously used in household paint and construction, which has been found to have harmful effects on humans, is _____lead_____

9. Bushes that adorn the front of homes are called _____shrubs_____

10. A face covering worn for disguise or performance is a _____mask_____

???

| FILL IN the BLANK to IDENTIFY a PLACE. Note: There may be more than one correct answer. |

1. A tropical location with heavy rainfall, dense undergrowth and millions of plants and insects is a

_____

2. The center of a hurricane is called its _____

3. The area of land used for takeoff and landing of aircraft is the _____

4. The large outdoor area where customers view movies from their cars is a _____

5. A building enclosed by glass or plastic and used to grow plants in all seasons is a _____

6. A facility used for overnight stay in a tent or recreational vehicle is a _____

7. The place where customers try on clothing in a department store is the _____

8. The playing area for tennis and basketball is a _____

9. Land overgrown with tangled vegetation is a _____

10. The point where an earthquake originates is called the

_____

```
┌─────────────────────────────┐
│        ANSWERS TO:          │
│   FILL IN the BLANK to      │
│   IDENTIFY a PLACE.         │
└─────────────────────────────┘
```

1. A tropical location with heavy rainfall, dense undergrowth and millions of plants and insects is a

   _____rainforest_____

2. The center of a hurricane is called its _____eye_____

3. The area of land used for takeoff and landing of aircraft is the _____runway_____

4. The large outdoor area where customers view movies from their cars is a _____drive-in_____

5. A building enclosed by glass or plastic and used to grow plants in all seasons is a ___greenhouse_____

6. A facility used for overnight stay in a tent or recreational vehicle is a _____campground_____

7. The place where customers try on clothing in a department store is the _____dressing room_____

8. The playing area for tennis and basketball is a _court_

9. Land overgrown with tangled vegetation is a _jungle_

10. The point where an earthquake originates is called the _____epicenter_____

??? Think about **TIME OR EVENTS** and **FILL IN** the **BLANK**. Note: There may be more than one correct answer.

1. When children spend the night at a friend's house, the special evening is called a _____

2. A treaty is typically signed by enemies at the end of a

   _____

3. Baseball games are divided into nine _____

4. The typical football game is divided into four, 15-minute _____

5. When a prisoner is restrained from contact with any others, he is placed in _____

6. A period of 100 years is termed a _____

7. A period of 10 years is a _____

8. A period of 1,000 years is a _____

9. The amount of time a prisoner must spend behind bars is called his or her _____

10. The provisional release of a prisoner who agrees to certain conditions is called a _____

> ## ANSWERS TO:
> Think about **TIME OR EVENTS** and **FILL IN** the **BLANK**.

1. When children spend the night at a friend's house, the special evening is called a ___sleepover___

2. A treaty is typically signed by enemies at the end of a ___war___

3. Baseball games are divided into nine ___innings___

4. The typical football game is divided into four, 15-minute ___quarters___

5. When a prisoner is restrained from contact with any others, he is placed in ___solitary confinement___

6. A period of 100 years is termed a ___century___

7. A period of 10 years is a ___decade___

8. A period of 1,000 years is a ___millenium___

9. The amount of time a prisoner must spend behind bars is called his or her ___sentence___

10. The provisional release of a prisoner who agrees to certain conditions is called ___parole or probation___

THINK ABOUT REASONS
WE DO THINGS and FILL IN
the BLANK. Note: There may be
more than one correct answer.

1. People who are very frightened might let out a _____

2. Pap smears and PSA tests are screenings for _____

3. Travelers use maps and GPS devices to be certain they are going in the right _____

4. When you discover a leaky faucet, you may need to replace the _____

5. To keep white clothing and linens free from stains, you might launder them with _____

6. Prisons are surrounded by wire, fencing and guard towers in order to prevent _____

7. People need to obtain a passport for travel _____

8. As cold, winter weather approaches, homeowners replace their screens with _____

9. People often begin a regimen of antibiotics when they have an _____

10. To be safe when riding in cars, passengers are advised to buckle their _____

ANSWERS TO:
THINK ABOUT REASONS
WE DO THINGS and FILL IN
the BLANK

1. People who are very frightened might let out a scream

2. Pap smears and PSA tests are screenings for cancer

3. Travelers use maps and GPS devices to be certain they are going in the right direction

4. When you discover a leaky faucet, you may need to replace the washer

5. To keep white clothing and linens free from stains, you might launder them with bleach

6. Prisons are surrounded by wire, fencing and guard towers in order to prevent escapes

7. People need to obtain a passport for travel abroad

8. As cold, winter weather approaches, homeowners replace their screens with storms

9. People often begin a regimen of antibiotics when they have an infection

10. To be safe when riding in cars, passengers are advised to buckle their seat belt

Printed in Great Britain
by Amazon.co.uk, Ltd.,
Marston Gate.